Fundamentals of Radiographic Positioning and Anatomy

T0337984

Fundamentals of Radiographic Positioning and Anatomy

JANE M. HARVEY-LLOYD
University of Leeds, Worsley Building,
Woodhouse, Leeds, UK, LS2 9TJ

RUTH M. STRUDWICK
University of Suffolk, H1.02, James Hehir Building,
University Avenue, Ipswich, UK, IP3 OFS

SCOTT J. PRESTON
The Open University, Walton Hall,
Milton Keynes, MK7 6AA

WILEY Blackwell

Registered Offices
John Wiley & Sons, Inc., 111 River Street, Hoboken, NJ 07030, USA
John Wiley & Sons Ltd, The Atrium, Southern Gate, Chichester, West Sussex, PO19 8SQ, UK

For details of our global editorial offices, customer services, and more information about Wiley products visit us at www.wiley.com.

Wiley also publishes its books in a variety of electronic formats and by print-on-demand. Some content that appears in standard print versions of this book may not be available in other formats.

Library of Congress Cataloging-in-Publication Data applied for
Paperback ISBN: 9781119826095

Cover Design: Wiley
Cover Image: © Peter Dazeley/Getty Images; serts/E+/Getty Images; LawrenceSawyer/Getty Images

Set in 9.5/12.5pt SourceSansPro by Straive, Chennai, India

Printed and bound in Great Britain by Bell & Bain Ltd, Glasgow

Contents

4 Shoulder Girdle   69

Clavicle
- Antero-posterior (AP) Projection of the Clavicle (Right)   **78**
- Infero-superior Projection of the Clavicle (Right)   **80**

5   Lower Limb   83

Hallux
- Dorsi-plantar (DP) Projection of the Hallux (Left)   **84**
- Lateral Projection of Hallux (Left)   **86**

Foot
- Dorsi-plantar (DP) Projection of the Foot (Left)   **88**
- Dorsi-plantar (DP) Oblique Projection of the Foot (Left)   **90**
- Turned Lateral Projection of the Foot (Left)   **92**

Calcaneum
- Axial Projection of the Calcaneum (Left)   **94**
- Lateral Projection of the Calcaneum (Left)   **96**

Ankle
- Antero-posterior (AP) Mortise Projection of the Ankle (Right)   **98**
- Lateral Projection of the Ankle (Right)   **100**

Tibia and Fibula
- Antero-posterior (AP) Projection of the Tibia and Fibula (Tib/Fib) (Left)   **102**
- Lateral Projection of the Tibia and Fibula (Tib/Fib) (Left)   **104**

Knee
- Antero-posterior Projection of the Knee (Left)   **106**
- Turned Lateral Projection of the Knee (Left)   **108**
- Horizontal Beam Lateral (HBL) Projection of the Knee (Right)   **110**

Femur
- Antero-posterior (AP) Projection of the Femur (Right) – Hip Down   **112**
- Antero-posterior (AP) Projection of the Femur (Right) – Knee Up   **114**

8 Skull and Facial Bones

Preface

This textbook was inspired by the original publication entitled *Basic Radiographic Positioning and Anatomy* by G.A. Bell and Dr D.B.L. Finlay. It is intended to be a useful, simple and practical guide for student radiographers, practitioners and educators by combining basic radiographic techniques with radiographic images and anatomical appearances.

The radiographic technique for each projection is described in a concise manner and accompanied by photographs demonstrating the patient positioning required. For each projection, a resultant radiograph is provided alongside a line drawing which outlines the anatomical appearances which can be seen on the radiograph. Space has been provided so you can personalise the textbook by completing the sections on common positioning faults and additional radiographic projections that can be undertaken. There is also an allocated 'other notes' section.

Diagnostic radiographers are a proud profession, and rightly so. The result of our work is often unseen by the patient and yet is crucial to patient care and their treatment pathway. We are, to many, 'invisible practitioners'. Thus, the knowledge and skills that go into producing a radiographic image can only truly be appreciated by those who have studied the science, informed by generations of research and experience.

We do hope that this textbook will help you to develop your knowledge and skills along your professional journey as a diagnostic radiographer.

Acknowledgements

Our thanks go to a range of staff from Buckinghamshire Healthcare NHS Trust: Jamie Sewell, (Senior Reporting Radiographer), Matt Wardlow (Radiology IT Manager) and Andrew Wainwright, (Head of Diagnostics) for the provision of the radiographic images. Also, thanks to Gemma Spelman, Lecturer at the University of Suffolk, for patiently and expertly editing the photographs and radiographic images used in this textbook, the University of Suffolk for the use of their imaging suite, Briony Leigh-Person, Lead Radiographer, Dental X-ray, East Suffolk and North Essex NHS Foundation Trust and the students from the University of Suffolk who gave their feedback on the initial ideas for the book.

Finally, our thanks goes to Charlie Harvey-Lloyd for demonstrating all the radiographic projections for the book in between studying for A-levels and his gymnastics training. I am sure you will agree, he was an excellent model!

CHAPTER 1

An Introduction to Radiographic Positioning and Terminology

This chapter will describe radiographic terminology in the following sections.

- Anatomical Terminology
- Positioning Terminology
- Projection Terminology
- Glossary of Terms

Fundamentals of Radiographic Positioning and Anatomy, First Edition.
Jane M. Harvey-Lloyd, Ruth M. Strudwick and Scott J. Preston.
© 2025 John Wiley & Sons Ltd. Published 2025 by John Wiley & Sons Ltd.

Anatomical Terminology

Diagnostic radiography uses a system of rules to describe the body and its movements. It is important to develop a good understanding of the terminology to be able to describe and understand the range of radiographic techniques outlined throughout this book. This terminology provides a clear and consistent approach to describing the location of anatomical structures and is used by a range of healthcare professionals. The use of this shared language enables clinicians and radiographers to communicate effectively in order to obtain the necessary diagnostic images.

The basic terminology descriptions refer to the standard reference position/orientation of the human body. This is known as the anatomical position.

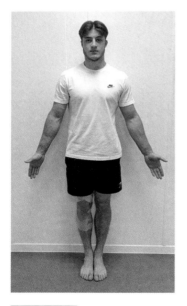

The standard anatomical position seen in Figure 1.1 can be described as a person in the following orientation.

- Standing upright and facing forward.
- Arms straight, hands at the level of the hips with palms facing forwards.
- Feet together with toes pointing forwards.

FIGURE 1.1 The anatomical position.

Using the anatomical position as the standard reference, the patient aspect can be described in the following terms.

Anterior aspect: this is seen when viewing the patient from the front.

Posterior aspect: this is seen when viewing the patient from the back.

Lateral aspect: this refers to any view of the patient (or any anatomical part) from the side e.g. the outer side of a limb.

Medial aspect: this refers to any view of the patient (or any anatomical part) which is closest to the midline, e.g. the inner side of a limb.

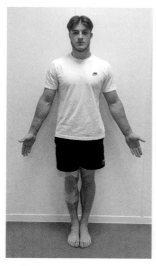 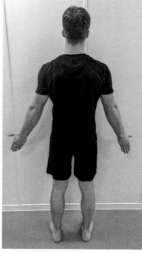 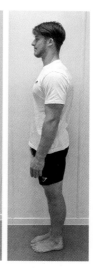

FIGURE 1.2 Anterior aspect.

FIGURE 1.3 Posterior aspect.

FIGURE 1.4 Lateral aspect.

Positioning Terminology

Planes of the Body

There are three planes of the body which are regularly used to describe the position of a patient in both projection and cross-sectional imaging.

Median sagittal plane: divides the body into equal left and right parts. Any plane parallel to this which divides the body into unequal right and left parts is known as a sagittal plane.

Coronal plane: divides the body into anterior and posterior parts.

Transverse/axial plane: divides the body into superior and inferior parts.

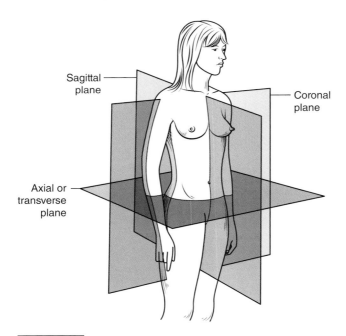

Sagittal plane

Coronal plane

Axial or transverse plane

FIGURE 1.5 Anatomical body planes.

Skull Positioning Lines and Planes

Skull, facial bone and dental radiography is undertaken with reference to recognised imaginary lines and planes of the skull. These assist radiographers (and others) when describing an area of interest or in positioning.

Lines of the Skull

- *Interpupillary (interorbital) line:* this is an imaginary line which joins the centre of the two pupils when the eyes are looking straight ahead.
- *Radiographic baseline (also known as the orbitomeatal line)*: this extends from the outer canthus of the eye on a slight diagonal line to the centre of the external auditory meatus (EAM).
- *Infraorbital line:* joins the two infraorbital points.
- *Anthropological baseline (also known as the Frankfurt line)*: passes from the infraorbital point to the upper border of the EAM.

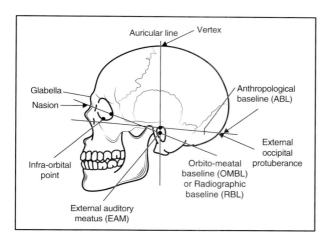

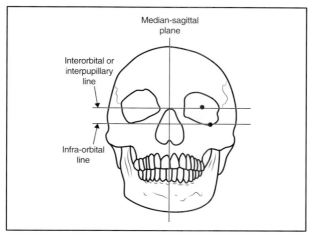

FIGURE 1.6 Anatomical positioning lines of the skull and face.

Planes of the Skull

- *Median sagittal plane*: divides the skull into equal left and right parts. Any plane parallel to this which divides the body into unequal right and left parts is known as a sagittal plane.
- *Coronal planes*: these run at right angles to the median sagittal plane and divide the head into anterior and posterior parts.
- *Transverse/axial plane*: divides the head into superior and inferior parts.
- *Auricular plane*: is perpendicular to the transverse/axial plane. It passes through the centre of the external auditory meatuses.

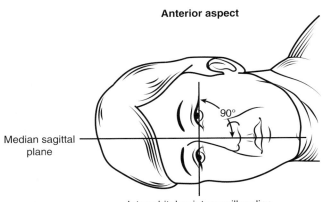

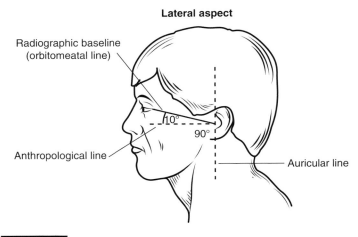

FIGURE 1.7 Planes of the skull.

Patient Positioning Terminology

The following terms are used to describe how the patient is positioned for a range of radiographic examinations/projections.

- *Erect*: the projection is taken with the patient either standing or sitting upright.
- *Decubitus*: the projection is taken with the patient lying down in any of the following positions.
  - Supine: the patient is lying on their back, face up.
  - Prone: the patient is lying on their front, and is face down.
  - Lateral decubitus: the patient is lying on their side. A right lateral decubitus is when the patient is lying on the right side; if the patient is facing the opposite side, this would be a left lateral decubitus.
  - Semi-recumbent: the patient is reclining, lying halfway between supine and sitting erect.

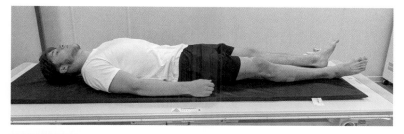

FIGURE 1.8 Supine.

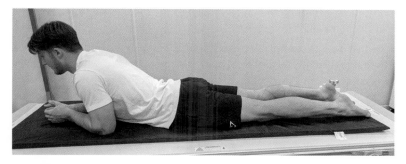

FIGURE 1.9 Prone.

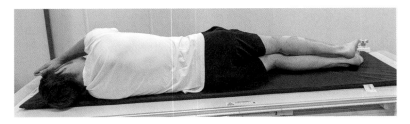

FIGURE 1.10 Lateral decubitus (left).

All these positions can be described more precisely by using a reference to the body planes, which ensures that the patient is accurately positioned, e.g. the patient is lying supine on the bed with the median sagittal plane at 90° to the image receptor (IR).

There are also some terms which are used to describe the anatomical position of the limbs which are explained in the Glossary of Terms at the end of this chapter.

Projection Terminology

A radiographic projection is described by the direction of the central ray in relation to the anatomical position and planes of the body.

Antero-posterior (AP): the central ray enters the anterior aspect of the body, passes through the body parallel to the median sagittal plane and exits from the posterior aspect.

Postero-anterior (PA): the central ray enters the posterior aspect of the body, passes through the body parallel to the median sagittal plane and exits from the anterior aspect.

Lateral (Lat): the central ray passes from one side of the body to the other, parallel to the coronal and axial planes. A right lateral is when the central ray enters the left aspect of the body and exits from the right side and vice versa for a left lateral.

Additional projection terminology, e.g. oblique, can be found in the Glossary of Terms.

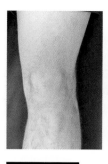

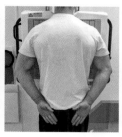

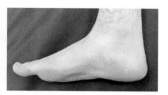

FIGURE 1.11 AP projection of the left knee.

FIGURE 1.12 PA projection of the chest.

FIGURE 1.13 Lateral projection of the foot (right).

To accurately describe a radiographic projection, the following should always be included.

- The position of the patient or area of interest in relation to the IR.
- The movements and degree of movement of the relevant joints, if appropriate.
- The direction and centring of the X-ray beam, e.g. a vertical central ray is centred to the lateral epicondyle
- The X-ray beam angulation relative to a starting point of vertical or horizontal.

In all the chapters, you will find that each radiographic projection has been described using this systematic approach.

Glossary of Terms

Abduct – to move a limb away from the middle of the body.

Adduct – to bring a limb toward the middle of the body.

Align – to place/arrange something in a straight line.

Anatomical position – a common visual reference point, with the person standing erect with feet together and eyes forward, palms face anteriorly with the thumbs pointed away from the body.

Anterior – towards or at the front.

Antero-posterior (AP) – term used to describe a radiographic projection in which the X-ray beam enters the anterior and then exits the posterior aspect of the body.

Artefact – something that appears on the resultant radiographic image that should not be there and detracts from the quality of the image. This could be caused by extraneous material on the patient or positioning aids or result from errors in the image processing.

Axial plane – an anatomical plane that divides the body into superior and inferior sections. Also known as the transverse plane.

Caudal – away from the head.

Contralateral – on the opposite side.

Coronal plane – a vertical plane running from side to side; divides the body or any of its parts into anterior and posterior portions.

Cranial – towards the head.

Decubitus – lying down.

Deep (internal) – away from the body surface.

Deviate – to move a part of the body out of its normal position, e.g. ulnar deviation

Distal – furthest from the origin or further from the point of attachment of a limb to the trunk.

Dorsum – the back or posterior surface, usually used for the hand or foot.

Elevate – to move something superiorly.

Elongation – where an object appears longer than it actually is on a radiographic image; this could be done intentionally to visualise a structure more clearly, e.g. in imaging the scaphoid.

Erect – sitting or standing upright.

Eversion – to move a joint outward or laterally.

Extension – straightening or extending a joint to increase the angle.

External – towards or at the body surface.

External auditory meatus (EAM) – the entrance point to the ear canal.

Flexion – bending or flexing a joint to decrease the angle.

Foreshortening – where an object appears shorter than it actually is on a radiographic image.

Frankfurt plane – a plane used in dental radiography which is a line passing from the lower border of the orbit to the external auditory meatus.

Fronto-occipital – term used to describe a radiographic projection of the skull/head in which the X-ray beam travels through the frontal bone and then the occiput bone.

Horizontal beam lateral (HBL) – a lateral projection in which the patient remains in a fixed position and the X-ray beam is directed with a horizontal beam to obtain a lateral projection.

Image receptor (IR) – the device used to capture the X-rays which pass through the patient to produce a radiograph.

Immobilise – to keep the area of the body being imaged still, which can be by way of equipment or by the patient holding their breath.

Inferior (caudal) – away from the head or toward the lower part of the structure or the body, e.g. the pelvis is inferior to the chest.

Internal – away from the body surface.

Interpupillary line – a line used in skull, facial bone and dental radiography which runs between the pupils of the eyes.

Inversion – to turn a joint inward or medially.

Ipsilateral – on the same side.

Lateral – away from the midline of the body.

Lateral decubitus – lying down on one side.

Medial – towards the middle of the body.

Median sagittal plane – a sagittal plane that bisects the body vertically through the midline, dividing the body exactly into equal left and right halves.

Object-to-image receptor distance (OID) – the distance between the object and the image receptor, affecting magnification.

Oblique – neither parallel nor at right angles to a specified or implied line; slanting.

Occipito-frontal – term used to describe a radiographic projection of the skull/head in which the X-ray beam enters through the occiput bone and exits through the frontal bone.

Occipito-mental – term used to describe a radiographic projection of the skull/head in which the X-ray beam enters through the occiput bone and exits through the symphysis menti of the mandible.

Palmar – the surface on the palm of the hand.

Palpate – examine a part of the body by touch, especially for medical purposes, e.g. positioning for an X-ray examination.

Plantar – the surface of the foot that is in contact with the floor when a person stands.

Posterior – towards or at the back.

Postero-anterior (PA) – term used to describe a radiographic projection in which the X-ray beam enters through the posterior and exits through the anterior aspect of the body.

Prone – lying on the front, face down.

Proximal – towards the origin or closer to the point of attachment of a limb to the trunk.

Radiographic baseline (RBL) – a line used in skull, facial bone and dental radiography which runs from the outer canthus to the external auditory meatus.

Radiolucent – permeable to radiation, such as X-rays. Radiolucent objects allow X-rays to pass through and therefore are not demonstrated on a radiographic image, e.g. air.

Radiopaque – opaque to radiation, such as X-rays. Radiopaque objects absorbs instead of block radiation rather than allow it to pass through and therefore are shown on a radiographic image, e.g. metal and bone.

Sagittal plane – a vertical plane which passes through the body longitudinally. It divides the body into a left section and a right section.

Semi-recumbent – between lying and sitting, an upright positioning of the head and torso at an angle of 45°.

Source-to-image receptor distance (SID) – the distance of the X-ray tube from the image receptor, affecting magnification. For most X-ray examinations, this is 100 cm.

Source-to-object distance (SOD) – the distance measured between the focal spot on the target of an X-ray tube and the centre mass of the patient's anatomical organ.

Superficial (external) – towards or at the body surface.

Superimpose – to place or lay a structure over another.

Superior (cranial) – towards the head or upper part of a structure or the body, e.g. the head is superior to the chest.

Supine – lying on the back facing upwards.

Transverse plane – an anatomical plane that divides the body into superior and inferior sections. Also known as the axial plane.

CHAPTER **2**

Thoracic Cavity and Abdomen

This chapter will cover all the routine radiographic projections under-taken of the thoracic cavity and abdomen. This will include the following projections.

- Chest
  - Postero-anterior (PA) Projection of the Chest
  - Lateral Projection of the Chest (Left)
- Sternum
  - Lateral Projection of the Sternum (Left)
- Abdomen
  - Antero-posterior (AP) Supine Projection of the Abdomen

Fundamentals of Radiographic Positioning and Anatomy, First Edition.
Jane M. Harvey-Lloyd, Ruth M. Strudwick and Scott J. Preston.
© 2025 John Wiley & Sons Ltd. Published 2025 by John Wiley & Sons Ltd.

Postero-anterior (PA) Projection of the Chest

Common Indications for Imaging

- Respiratory tract infections
- Pneumonia
- Pneumothorax
- Inhaled or aspirated foreign body
- Shortness of breath

Radiographic Technique

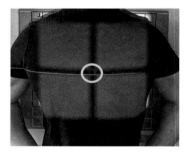

FIGURE 2.1 Patient positioning for the PA chest projection.

- Stand the patient erect facing the IR with their feet apart and the anterior part of their chest in contact with the IR.
- Place the dorsal surface of the patient's hands on the hips.
- Move the shoulders and humeri anteriorly, to clear the scapulae from the lung fields.
- Ensure that the median sagittal plane is perpendicular to the IR and the patient is not rotated.
- Place the anatomical marker in the primary beam.
- Collimate to include superiorly from the apices to the bases of the lungs inferiorly and the skin borders laterally.
- The exposure should be made on arrested inspiration.

Centring point: with a horizontal central ray at 90° to the IR at the level of the spinous process of the sixth thoracic vertebra in the midline.

Radiographic Anatomy

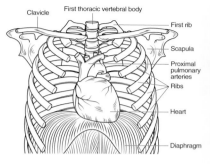

Clavicle
First thoracic vertebral body
First rib
Scapula
Proximal pulmonary arteries
Ribs
Heart
Diaphragm

FIGURE 2.2   Anatomy of the PA chest projection.

Resultant Image

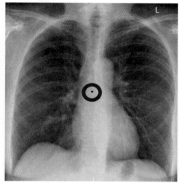

L

FIGURE 2.3   Resultant image of the PA chest projection.

Common positioning faults:

Additional projections:

Other notes:

Lateral Projection of the Chest (Left)

Common Indications for Imaging

- Location or size of tumour, infection or consolidation
- Position of pacemaker wires

Radiographic Technique

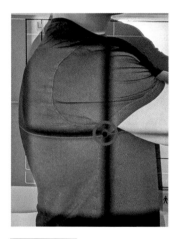

FIGURE 2.4 Patient positioning for the left lateral projection of the chest.

- Stand the patient in the true lateral position with their feet apart so that the left side of the patient's chest is in contact with the IR.
- Raise the arms away from the chest.
- Ensure that the median sagittal plane is parallel to the IR and the patient is not rotated.
- Place the left anatomical marker in the primary beam.
- Collimate to include superiorly from the apices to the bases of the lungs inferiorly and the skin borders laterally.
- The exposure should be made on arrested inspiration.

Centring point: with a horizontal central ray at 90° to the IR to the right axilla.

Radiographic Anatomy

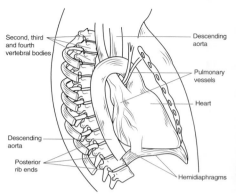

Second, third and fourth vertebral bodies

Descending aorta

Pulmonary vessels

Heart

Descending aorta

Posterior rib ends

Hemidiaphragms

FIGURE 2.5   Anatomy of the left lateral projection of the chest.

Resultant Image

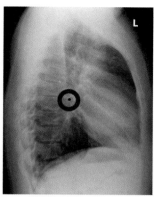

FIGURE 2.6   Resultant image of the left lateral projection of the chest.

Common positioning faults:

Additional projections:

Other notes:

Lateral Projection of the Sternum (Left)

Common Indications for Imaging

- Fractures of sternum

Radiographic Technique

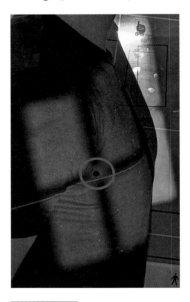

- Stand the patient in the true lateral position with their feet apart so that the left side of the patient's chest is in contact with the IR.
- Move the shoulders back and away from the chest, placing the hands behind the back.
- Ensure that the median sagittal plane is parallel to the IR and the patient is not rotated.
- Place the left anatomical marker in the primary beam.
- Collimate to include the sternum.
- The exposure should be made on arrested inspiration.

FIGURE 2.7 Patient positioning for the left lateral projection of the sternum.

Centring point: with a horizontal central ray at 90° to the IR to the sternal angle.

Radiographic Anatomy

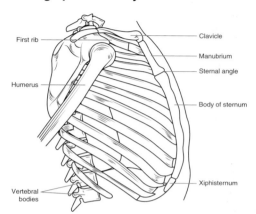

First rib
Clavicle
Manubrium
Sternal angle
Humerus
Body of sternum
Vertebral bodies
Xiphisternum

FIGURE 2.8   Anatomy for the left lateral projection of the sternum.

Resultant Image

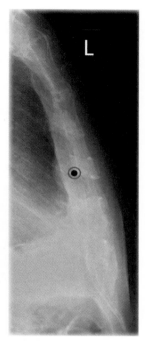

L

FIGURE 2.9   Resultant image of the left lateral projection of the sternum.

Common positioning faults:

Additional projections:

Other notes:

Antero-posterior (AP) Supine Projection of the Abdomen

Common Indications for Imaging

- Acute pain
- Renal colic and renal calculi
- Bowel obstruction

Radiographic Technique

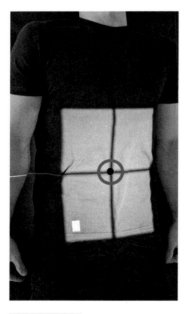

- Lie the patient supine on the table.
- Ensure that the median sagittal plane is parallel to the tabletop and perpendicular to the IR.
- Ensure that the patient is not rotated, and the anterior superior iliac spines (ASIS) are equidistant from the IR.
- Place the anatomical marker in the primary beam.
- Collimate to include the diaphragm superiorly, the symphysis pubis inferiorly and the skin borders laterally.
- The exposure should be made on arrested expiration.

FIGURE 2.10 Patient positioning for the AP abdomen projection.

Centring point: with a vertical central ray at 90° to the IR in the midline at the level of the iliac crests.

Radiographic Anatomy

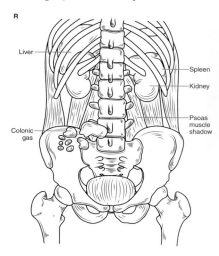

R

Liver

Spleen

Kidney

Psoas
muscle
shadow

Colonic
gas

FIGURE 2.11   Anatomy of the AP
abdomen projection.

Resultant Image

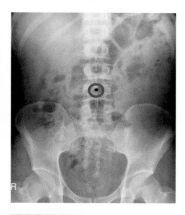

R

FIGURE 2.12   Resultant image of
the AP abdomen projection.

Common positioning faults:

Additional projections:

Other notes:

CHAPTER **3**

Upper Limb

This chapter will cover all the routine radiographic projections undertaken of the upper limb. This will include the following projections.

- Fingers
  - Dorsi-palmar (DP) Projection of the Index and Middle Fingers (Left)
  - Lateral Projection of the Index Finger (Left)
  - Lateral Projection of the Middle Finger (Left)
  - Dorsi-palmar (DP) Projection of the Ring and Little Fingers (Left)
  - Lateral Projection of the Ring Finger (Left)
  - Lateral Projection of the Little Finger (Left)
- Thumb
  - Antero-posterior (AP) Projection of the Thumb (Right)
  - Postero-anterior (PA) Projection of the Thumb (Right)
  - Lateral Projection of the Thumb (Right)
- Hand
  - Dorsi-palmar (DP) Projection of the Hand (Left)
  - Dorsi-palmar (DP) Oblique Projection of the Hand (Left)
  - Lateral Projection of the Hand (Left)
- Wrist
  - Postero-anterior (PA) Projection of the Wrist (Right)
  - Lateral Projection of the Wrist (Right)
- Scaphoid
  - Postero-anterior (PA) Oblique Projection with Ulnar Deviation of the Wrist for Scaphoid (Left)
  - Zitter's Projection of the Wrist for Scaphoid (Left)
- Forearm
  - Antero-posterior (AP) Projection of the Forearm (Right)
  - Lateral Projection of the Forearm (Right)
- Elbow
  - Antero-posterior (AP) Projection of the Elbow (Right)
  - Lateral Projection of the Elbow (Right)
- Humerus
  - Antero-posterior (AP) Projection of the Humerus (Left)
  - Lateral Projection of the Humerus (Left)

Fundamentals of Radiographic Positioning and Anatomy, First Edition.
Jane M. Harvey-Lloyd, Ruth M. Strudwick and Scott J. Preston.
© 2025 John Wiley & Sons Ltd. Published 2025 by John Wiley & Sons Ltd.

Dorsi-palmar (DP) Projection of the Index and Middle Fingers (Left)

Common Indications for Imaging

- Fractures of base of first metacarpal
- Fractures of metacarpals and phalanges
- Dislocation of interphalangeal joint
- Dislocation of metacarpal joint
- Salter Harris fracture

Radiographic Technique

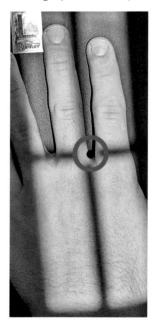

FIGURE 3.1   Patient positioning for the DP projection of the left index and middle fingers.

- Seat the patient with the affected side nearest the IR.
- Extend the patient's hand and wrist then flex the elbow so that the palmar aspect of the hand is in contact with the IR.
- Extend the patient's fingers and separate them slightly whilst spacing evenly.
- Place the left anatomical marker in the primary beam – in this case on the left side of the left index and middle fingers.
- Collimate to include from the distal phalanx to the metacarpal joint, including the index and middle fingers laterally and medially respectively for orientation purposes.

Centring point: with a vertical central ray at 90° to the IR to the proximal interphalangeal joint of the affected finger.

Radiographic Anatomy

L

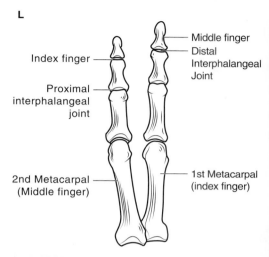

Index finger

Middle finger

Distal Interphalangeal Joint

Proximal interphalangeal joint

2nd Metacarpal (Middle finger)

1st Metacarpal (index finger)

FIGURE 3.2 Anatomy of the DP projection of the left index and middle fingers.

Resultant Image

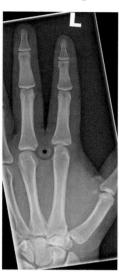

FIGURE 3.3 Resultant image of the DP projection of the left index and middle fingers.

Common positioning faults:	Other notes:
Additional projections:	

Lateral Projection of the Index Finger (Left)

Common Indications for Imaging

- Fractures of base of first metacarpal
- Fractures of metacarpals and phalanges
- Dislocation of interphalangeal joint
- Dislocation of metacarpal joint
- Salter Harris fractures

Radiographic Technique

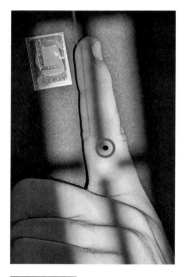

FIGURE 3.4   Patient positioning of the lateral projection of left index finger.

- Seat the patient with the affected side nearest the IR.
- Extend the patient's hand and wrist then flex the elbow so that the palmar aspect of the hand is in contact with the IR.
- Rotate the hand medially and place the lateral aspect of the index finger so that it is in contact with the IR and then flex the other fingers.
- Place the left anatomical marker in the primary beam – in this case on the left side of the left index finger.
- Collimate to include from the distal phalanx to the metacarpal joint.

Centring point: with a vertical central ray at 90° to the IR to the proximal interphalangeal joint of the left index finger.

Radiographic Anatomy

L

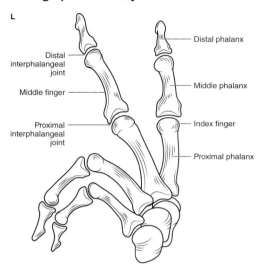

Distal phalanx

Distal interphalangeal joint

Middle finger

Proximal interphalangeal joint

Middle phalanx

Index finger

Proximal phalanx

FIGURE 3.5 Anatomy of the lateral projection of left index finger.

Resultant Image

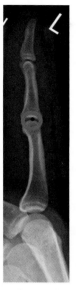

FIGURE 3.6 Resultant image of the lateral projection of left index finger.

Common positioning faults:

Additional projections:

Other notes:

Lateral Projection of the Middle Finger (Left)

Common Indications for Imaging

- Fractures of base of first metacarpal
- Fractures of metacarpals and phalanges
- Dislocation of interphalangeal joint
- Dislocation of metacarpal joint
- Salter Harris fractures

Radiographic Technique

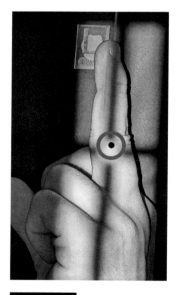

- Seat the patient with the affected side nearest the IR.
- Extend the patient's hand and wrist then flex the elbow so that the palmar aspect of the hand is in contact with the IR.
- Rotate the hand medially and place the middle finger parallel to the IR; flex the other fingers.
- Place the right anatomical marker in the primary beam – in this case on the left side of the left middle finger.
- Collimate to include from the distal phalanx to the metacarpal joint.

FIGURE 3.7 Patient positioning for the lateral projection of the left middle finger.

Centring point: with a vertical central ray at 90° to the IR to the proximal interphalangeal joint of the left middle finger.

Radiographic Anatomy

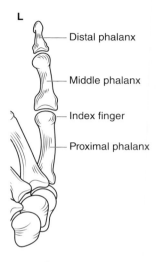

L

Distal phalanx

Middle phalanx

Index finger

Proximal phalanx

FIGURE 3.8 Anatomy of the lateral projection of the left middle finger.

Resultant Image

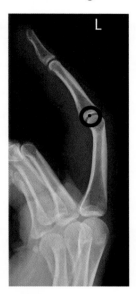

FIGURE 3.9 Resultant image of the lateral projection of the left middle finger.

Common positioning faults:

Additional projections:

Other notes:

Dorsi-palmar (DP) Projection of the Ring and Little Fingers (Left)

Common Indications for Imaging

- Fractures of base of first metacarpal
- Fractures of metacarpals and phalanges
- Dislocation of interphalangeal joint
- Dislocation of metacarpal joint
- Salter Harris fractures

Radiographic Technique

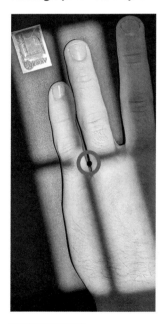

- Seat the patient with the affected side nearest the IR.
- Extend the patient's hand and wrist then flex the elbow so that the palmar aspect of the hand is in contact with the IR.
- Extend the patient's fingers and separate them slightly whilst spacing evenly.
- Place the left anatomical marker in the primary beam – in this case on the left side of the left fingers.
- Collimate to include from the distal phalanx to the metacarpal joint, including an adjacent finger laterally or medially for orientation purposes.

FIGURE 3.10 Patient positioning for the DP projection of the left ring and little fingers.

Centring point: with a vertical central ray at 90° to the IR to the proximal interphalangeal joint of the affected finger.

Radiographic Anatomy

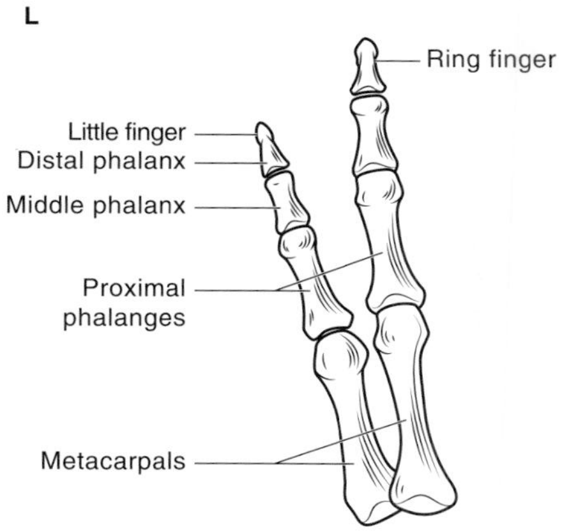

L

Ring finger

Little finger
Distal phalanx
Middle phalanx

Proximal
phalanges

Metacarpals

FIGURE 3.11 Anatomy of the DP projection of the left ring and little fingers.

Resultant Image

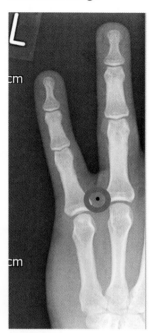

FIGURE 3.12 Resultant image of the DP projection of the right ring and little fingers.

Common positioning faults:

Additional projections:

Other notes:

Lateral Projection of the Ring Finger (Left)

Common Indications for Imaging

- Fractures of base of first metacarpal
- Fractures of metacarpals and phalanges
- Dislocation of interphalangeal joint
- Dislocation of metacarpal joint
- Salter Harris fractures

Radiographic Technique

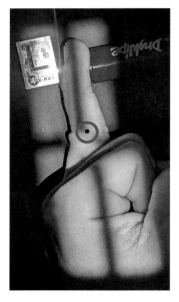

- Seat the patient with the affected side nearest the IR.
- Extend the patient's hand and wrist then flex the elbow so that the palmar aspect of the hand is in contact with the IR.
- Rotate the hand laterally and place the medial aspect of the ring finger parallel to the IR; flex the other fingers.
- Place the left anatomical marker in the primary beam – in this case on the left side of the left ring finger.
- Collimate to include from the distal phalanx to the metacarpal joint.

FIGURE 3.13 Patient positioning for the lateral projection of the left ring finger.

Centring point: with a vertical central ray at 90° to the IR to the proximal interphalangeal joint of the left ring finger.

Radiographic Anatomy

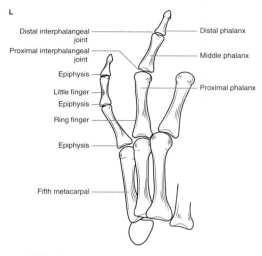

L

Distal interphalangeal joint

Proximal interphalangeal joint

Epiphysis

Little finger

Epiphysis

Ring finger

Epiphysis

Fifth metacarpal

Distal phalanx

Middle phalanx

Proximal phalanx

FIGURE 3.14   Anatomy of the lateral projection of the left ring finger.

Resultant Image

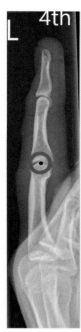

FIGURE 3.15   Resultant image of the lateral projection of the left ring finger.

Common positioning faults:
Additional projections:

Other notes:

Lateral Projection of the Little Finger (Left)

Common Indications for Imaging

- Fractures of base of first metacarpal
- Fractures of metacarpals and phalanges
- Dislocation of interphalangeal joint
- Dislocation of metacarpal joint
- Salter Harris fracture

Radiographic Technique

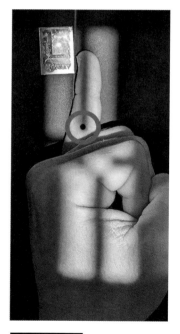

- Seat the patient with the affected side nearest the IR.
- Extend the patient's hand and wrist then flex the elbow so that the palmar aspect of the hand is in contact with the IR.
- Rotate the hand laterally and place the medial aspect of the little finger so that it is in contact with the IR and flex the other fingers.
- Place the left anatomical marker in the primary beam – in this case on the left side of the left little finger.
- Collimate to include from the distal phalanx to the metacarpal joint.

FIGURE 3.16 Patient positioning for the lateral projection of the left little finger.

Centring point: with a vertical central ray at 90° to the IR to the proximal interphalangeal joint of the affected finger.

Radiographic Anatomy

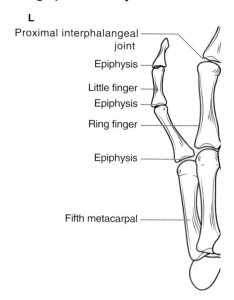

L
Proximal interphalangeal joint
Epiphysis
Little finger
Epiphysis
Ring finger
Epiphysis
Fifth metacarpal

FIGURE 3.17   Anatomy of the lateral projection of the left little finger.

Resultant Image

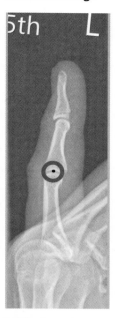

FIGURE 3.18   Resultant image of the lateral projection of the left little finger.

Common positioning faults:

Additional projections:

Other notes:

Antero-posterior (AP) Projection of the Thumb (Right)

Common Indications for Imaging

- Bennett's fracture
- Fractures of metacarpals and phalanges
- Osteoarthritis

Radiographic Technique

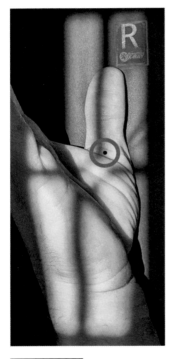

- Seat the patient with the affected side nearest the IR.
- Extend the patient's hand, wrist and elbow.
- Medially rotate the arm until the posterior aspect of the thumb is in contact with the IR.
- Place the right anatomical marker in the primary beam – in this case on the right side of the right thumb.
- Collimate to include from the distal phalanx to the meta-carpal joint.

FIGURE 3.19 Patient positioning for the AP projection of the right thumb.

Centring point: with a vertical central ray at 90° to the IR to the metacar-pophalangeal joint of the right thumb.

Radiographic Anatomy

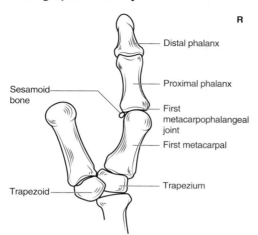

R

- Distal phalanx
- Proximal phalanx

Sesamoid bone

- First metacarpophalangeal joint
- First metacarpal

Trapezoid

- Trapezium

FIGURE 3.20   Anatomy of the AP projection of the right thumb.

Resultant Image

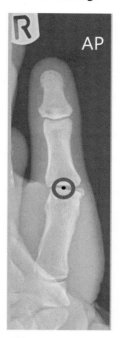

R

AP

FIGURE 3.21   Resultant image of the AP projection of the right thumb.

Common positioning faults:

Additional projections:

Other notes:

Postero-anterior (PA) Projection of the Thumb (Right)

Common Indications for Imaging

- Fractures of base of first metacarpal
- Fractures of metacarpals and phalanges
- Osteoarthritis
- Rheumatoid arthritis

Radiographic Technique

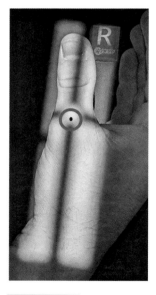

- Seat the patient with the affected side nearest the IR.
- Extend the patient's hand and wrist then flex the elbow and place the medial aspect of the hand in contact with the IR.
- Extend the patient's thumb and rest it on a small radiolucent pad (if needed).
- Place the right anatomical marker in the primary beam – in this case on the right side of the right thumb.
- Collimate to include from the distal phalanx to the metacarpal joint.

FIGURE 3.22 Patient positioning for the PA projection of the right thumb.

Centring point: with a vertical central ray at 90° to the IR to the metacarpophalangeal joint of the right thumb.

Radiographic Anatomy

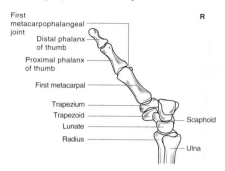

First metacarpophalangeal joint

Distal phalanx of thumb

Proximal phalanx of thumb

First metacarpal

Trapezium

Trapezoid

Lunate

Radius

R

Scaphoid

Ulna

FIGURE 3.23 Anatomy of the PA projection of the right thumb.

Resultant Image

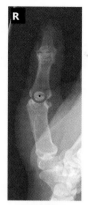

R

FIGURE 3.24 Resultant image of the PA projection of the right thumb. This radiograph/image demonstrates a pathology/condition which will not always be present. It has been included here to demonstrate the ideal positioning and exposure.

Common positioning faults:

Additional projections:

Other notes:

Lateral Projection of the Thumb (Right)

Common Indications for Imaging

- Bennett's fracture
- Fractures of metacarpals and phalanges
- Osteoarthritis

Radiographic Technique

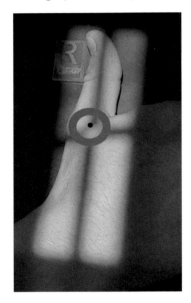

- Seat the patient with the affected side nearest the IR.
- Extend the patient's hand and wrist then flex the elbow so that the palmar aspect of the hand is in contact with the IR.
- Separate the thumb and rotate the hand so that the lateral border of the thumb is in contact with the IR.
- Place the right anatomical marker in the primary beam – in this case on the right side of the right thumb.
- Collimate to include from the distal phalanx to the metacarpal joint.

FIGURE 3.25 Patient positioning for the lateral projection of the right thumb.

Centring point: with a vertical central ray at 90° to the IR to the metacarpophalangeal joint of the right thumb.

Radiographic Anatomy

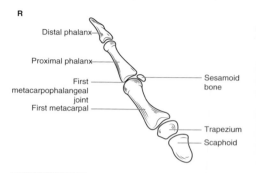

R

Distal phalanx

Proximal phalanx

First
metacarpophalangeal
joint

First metacarpal

Sesamoid
bone

Trapezium

Scaphoid

FIGURE 3.26   Anatomy of the lateral projection of the right thumb.

Resultant Image

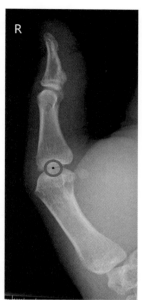

R

FIGURE 3.27   Resultant image of the lateral projection of the right thumb.

Common positioning faults:

Additional projections:

Other notes:

Dorsi-palmar (DP) Projection of the Hand (Left)

Common Indications for Imaging

- Fractures of base of first metacarpal
- Fractures of metacarpals and phalanges
- Osteoarthritis
- Rheumatoid arthritis

Radiographic Technique

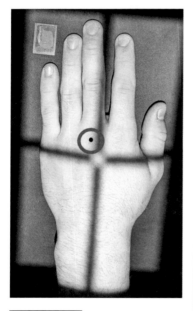

- Seat the patient with the affected side nearest the IR.
- Extend the patient's hand and wrist then flex the elbow so that the palmar aspect of the hand is in contact with the IR.
- Extend the patient's fingers and separate them slightly whilst spacing evenly.
- Place the left anatomical marker in the primary beam – in this case on the left side of the left hand.
- Collimate to include the distal third of the forearm, the distal phalanges and the lateral borders of the hand.

FIGURE 3.28 Patient positioning for the DP projection of the left hand.

Centring point: with a vertical central ray at 90° to the IR at the head of the third metacarpal of the left hand.

Radiographic Anatomy

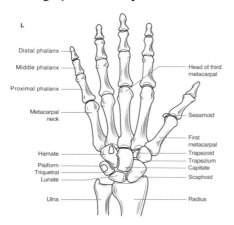

FIGURE 3.29   Anatomy of the DP projection of the left hand.

Resultant Image

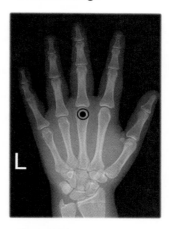

FIGURE 3.30   Resultant image of the DP projection of the left hand.

Common positioning faults:

Additional projections:

Other notes:

Dorsi-palmar (DP) Oblique Projection of the Hand (Left)

Common Indications for Imaging

- Fractures of base of first metacarpal
- Fractures of metacarpals and phalanges
- Osteoarthritis
- Rheumatoid arthritis

Radiographic Technique

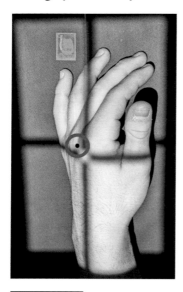

FIGURE 3.31 Patient positioning for the DP oblique projection of the left hand.

- Seat the patient with the affected side nearest the IR.
- Extend the patient's hand and wrist then flex the elbow so that the palmar aspect of the hand is in contact with the IR.
- Externally rotate the wrist and rest the patient's thumb on the IR so that the palmar aspect of the hand is at 45° to the IR.
- Extend the patient's fingers and separate them slightly whilst spacing evenly.
- Place the left anatomical marker in the primary beam – in this case on the left side of the left hand.
- Collimate to include the distal third of the forearm, the distal phalanges and the lateral borders of the hand.

Centring point: with a vertical central ray at 90° to the IR at the head of the fifth metacarpal of the left hand.

Radiographic Anatomy

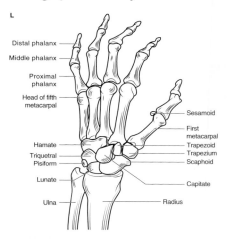

L

Distal phalanx
Middle phalanx
Proximal phalanx
Head of fifth metacarpal

Sesamoid
First metacarpal
Hamate — Trapezoid
Triquetral — Trapezium
Pisiform — Scaphoid
Lunate
Capitate
Ulna — Radius

FIGURE 3.32 Anatomy of the DP oblique projection of the left hand.

Resultant Image

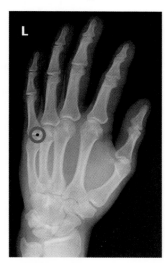

FIGURE 3.33 Resultant image of the DP oblique projection of the left hand.

Common positioning faults:

Additional projections:

Other notes:

Lateral Projection of the Hand (Left)

Common Indications for Imaging

- Displaced fractures of metacarpals and phalanges
- Location of foreign body

Radiographic Technique

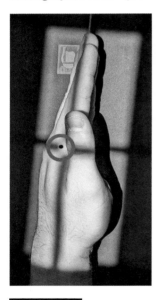

FIGURE 3.34 Patient positioning for the lateral projection of the left hand.

- Seat the patient with the affected side nearest the IR.
- Extend the patient's hand and wrist then flex the elbow so that the palmar aspect of the hand is in contact with the IR.
- Externally rotate the wrist, so that the medial aspect of the hand is in contact with the IR, and extend the fingers.
- Place the left anatomical marker in the primary beam – in this case on the left side of the left hand.
- Collimate to include the distal third of the forearm, the distal phalanges and the palmar and dorsal borders of the hand.

Centring point: with a vertical central ray at 90° to the IR at the proximal interphalangeal joint of the index finger of the left hand.

Radiographic Anatomy

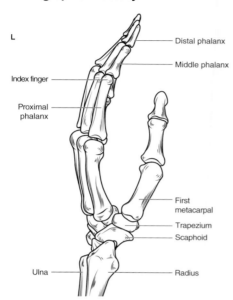

L

Index finger

Proximal phalanx

Ulna

Distal phalanx

Middle phalanx

First metacarpal

Trapezium

Scaphoid

Radius

FIGURE 3.35 Anatomy of the lateral projection of the left hand.

Resultant Image

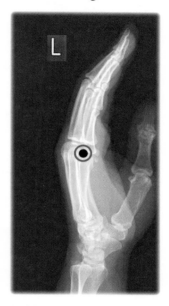

FIGURE 3.36 Resultant image of the lateral projection of the left hand.

Common positioning faults:

Additional projections:

Other notes:

Postero-anterior (PA) Projection of the Wrist (Right)

Common Indications for Imaging

- Fractures of the wrist joint, e.g. Colles' fracture or Smith's fracture
- Fractures of the distal radius and ulna
- Osteoarthritis
- Rheumatoid arthritis
- Dislocation of wrist joint or carpal bones

Radiographic Technique

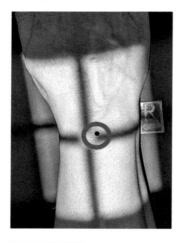

FIGURE 3.37   Patient positioning for the PA projection of the right wrist.

- Seat the patient with the affected side nearest the IR.
- Extend the patient's hand and wrist then flex the elbow so that the anterior aspect of the wrist is in contact with the IR.
- Ask the patient to make a fist or place a foam pad under the metacarpophalangeal joints to maintain the wrist in close contact with the IR.
- Place the right anatomical marker in the primary beam – in this case on the right side of the right wrist.
- Collimate to include the distal third of the forearm, the metacarpals and the lateral borders of the wrist.

Centring point: with a vertical central ray at 90° to the IR to a point midway between the radial and ulnar styloid processes of the right wrist.

Radiographic Anatomy

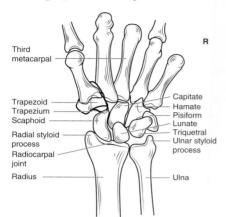

Third metacarpal

Trapezoid
Trapezium
Scaphoid
Radial styloid process
Radiocarpal joint
Radius

Capitate
Hamate
Pisiform
Lunate
Triquetral
Ulnar styloid process

Ulna

R

FIGURE 3.38   Anatomy of the PA projection of the right wrist.

Resultant Image

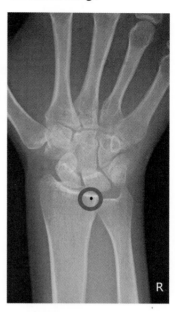

R

FIGURE 3.39   Resultant image of the PA projection of the right wrist.

Common positioning faults:

Additional projections:

Other notes:

Lateral Projection of the Wrist (Right)

Common Indications for Imaging

- Fractures of the wrist joint, e.g. Colles' fracture or Smith's fracture
- Fractures of the distal radius and ulna
- Osteoarthritis
- Rheumatoid arthritis
- Dislocation of wrist joint or carpal bones

Radiographic Technique

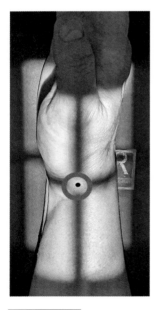

FIGURE 3.40 Patient positioning for the lateral projection of the right wrist.

- Seat the patient with the affected side nearest the IR.
- Extend the patient's hand and wrist, flex the elbow and rotate the patient's wrist so that the fifth finger and medial aspect of the forearm are in contact with the IR.
- Ensure that the radial and ulnar styloid processes are superimposed.
- Place the right anatomical marker in the primary beam – in this case on the right side of the right wrist.
- Collimate to include the distal third of the forearm, the metacarpals and the lateral borders of the wrist.

Centring point: with a vertical central ray at 90° to the IR to the radial styloid process.

Radiographic Anatomy

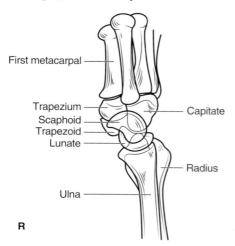

First metacarpal

Trapezium
Scaphoid
Trapezoid
Lunate

Capitate

Radius

Ulna

R

FIGURE 3.41   Anatomy of the lateral projection of the right wrist.

Resultant Image

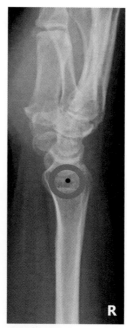

R

FIGURE 3.42   Resultant image of the lateral projection of the right wrist.

Common positioning faults:

Additional projections:

Other notes:

Postero-anterior (PA) Oblique Projection with Ulnar Deviation of the Wrist for Scaphoid (Left)

Common Indications for Imaging

- Fracture of scaphoid

Radiographic Technique

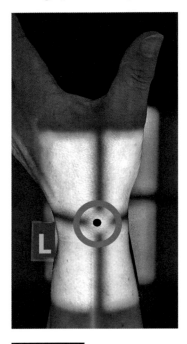

- Seat the patient with the affected side nearest the IR.
- Extend the patient's hand and wrist then flex the elbow so that the anterior aspect of the wrist is in contact with the IR with ulnar deviation of the wrist.
- Rotate the wrist laterally so that the palmar aspect is at 45° to the IR.
- Place the left anatomical marker in the primary beam – in this case on the left side of the left wrist.
- Collimate to include the distal third of the forearm, the metacarpals and the lateral borders of the scaphoid.

FIGURE 3.43   Patient positioning for the PA oblique projection with ulnar deviation of the left wrist.

Centring point: with a vertical central ray at 90° to the IR to a point midway between the radial and ulnar styloid processes of the left wrist.

Radiographic Anatomy

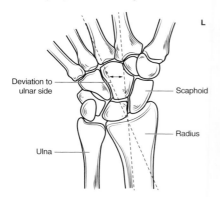

FIGURE 3.44   Anatomy of the PA oblique projection with ulnar deviation of the left wrist

Resultant Image

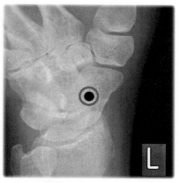

FIGURE 3.45   Resultant image of the PA oblique projection with ulnar deviation of the left wrist.

Common positioning faults:

Additional projections:

Other notes:

Zitter's Projection of the Wrist for Scaphoid (Left)

Common Indications for Imaging

- Fracture of scaphoid

Radiographic Technique

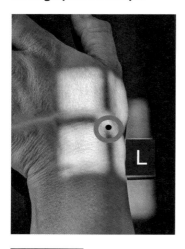

FIGURE 3.46 Patient positioning for the Zitter's projection of the left wrist.

- Seat the patient with the affected side nearest the IR.
- Extend the patient's hand and wrist then flex the elbow so that the anterior aspect of the wrist is in contact with the IR.
- Ask the patient to move their wrist into ulnar deviation.
- Place the left anatomical marker in the primary beam – in this case on the left side of the left wrist.
- Collimate to include the scaphoid.

Centring point: with a vertical central ray with the X-ray tube angled 30° towards the head (cranially), centred over the anatomical snuff box of the left wrist.

Radiographic Anatomy

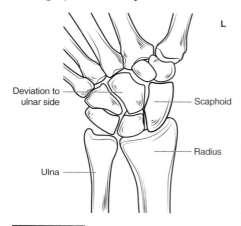

L

FIGURE 3.47   Anatomy of the Zitter's projection of the left wrist.

Resultant Image

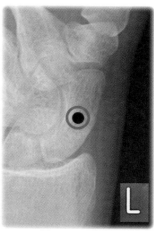

FIGURE 3.48   Resultant image of the Zitter's projection of the left wrist.

Common positioning faults:

Additional projections:

Other notes:

Antero-posterior (AP) Projection of the Forearm (Right)

Common Indications for Imaging

- Fractures of midshaft radius and ulna
- Monteggia's fracture-dislocation
- Galeazzi fracture-dislocation

Radiographic Technique

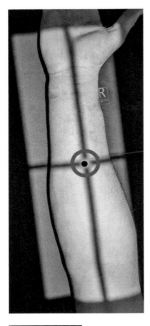

FIGURE 3.49 Patient positioning for the AP projection of the right forearm.

- Seat the patient with the affected side nearest the IR.
- Extend the patient's arm, so that the elbow and wrist are extended and in the same plane and the posterior aspect of the forearm is in contact with the IR.
- The radial and ulnar styloid processes should be equidistant from the IR and the medial and lateral epicondyles should also be equidistant from the IR.
- Place the right anatomical marker in the primary beam – in this case on the right side of the right forearm.
- Collimate to include the wrist joint, the elbow joint and the lateral borders of the forearm.

Centring point: with a vertical central ray at 90° to the IR to midpoint of the shaft of the radius and ulna of the right forearm.

Radiographic Anatomy

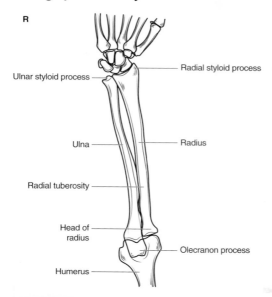

R

Ulnar styloid process

Radial styloid process

Ulna — Radius

Radial tuberosity

Head of radius

Olecranon process

Humerus

FIGURE 3.50 Anatomy of the AP projection of the right forearm.

Resultant Image

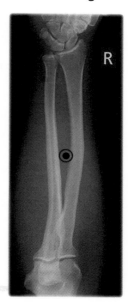

R

FIGURE 3.51 Resultant image of the AP projection of the right forearm.

Common positioning faults:

Additional projections:

Other notes:

Lateral Projection of the Forearm (Right)

Common Indications for Imaging

- Fractures of midshaft radius and ulna
- Monteggia's fracture-dislocation
- Galeazzi fracture-dislocation

Radiographic Technique

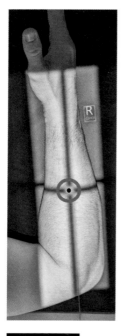

- Seat the patient with the affected side nearest the IR.
- Flex the elbow to 90° and rotate the forearm to the true lateral position with the thumb uppermost.
- Ensure that the medial aspect of the forearm is in contact with the IR.
- The radial and ulnar styloid processes should be superimposed.
- Place the right anatomical marker in the primary beam – in this case on the right side of the right forearm.
- Collimate to include the wrist joint, the elbow joint and the lateral borders of the forearm.

FIGURE 3.52 Patient positioning for the lateral projection of the right forearm.

Centring point: with a vertical central ray at 90° to the IR to midpoint of the shaft of the radius and ulna.

Radiographic Anatomy

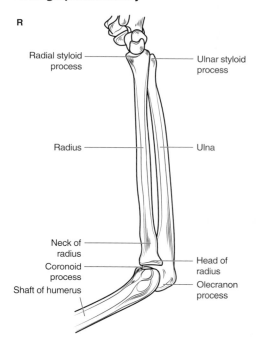

R

Radial styloid process

Ulnar styloid process

Radius

Ulna

Neck of radius

Coronoid process

Head of radius

Shaft of humerus

Olecranon process

FIGURE 3.53 Anatomy of the lateral forearm projection.

Resultant Image

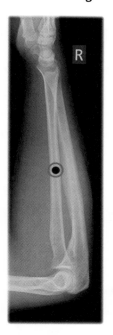

FIGURE 3.54 Resultant image of the lateral forearm projection.

Common positioning faults:

Additional projections:

Other notes:

Antero-posterior (AP) Projection of the Elbow (Right)

Common Indications for Imaging

- Fracture of the olecranon process, radial head, distal humerus, e.g. supracondylar fracture
- Dislocation of the elbow
- Osteoarthritis

Radiographic Technique

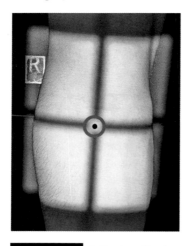

FIGURE 3.55 Patient positioning for the AP projection of the right elbow.

- Seat the patient with the affected side nearest the IR.
- Extend the patient's arm, so that the wrist, elbow and shoulder are extended and in the same plane, the arm is fully supinated and the posterior aspect of the forearm and humerus is in contact with the IR.
- The medial and lateral epicondyles should also be equidistant from the IR.
- Place the right anatomical marker in the primary beam – in this case on the right side of the right elbow.
- Collimate to include the proximal third of the forearm, the distal third of the humerus and the lateral borders of the elbow.

Centring point: with a vertical central ray at 90° to the IR to a point midway between the medial and lateral epicondyles of the right humerus.

Radiographic Anatomy

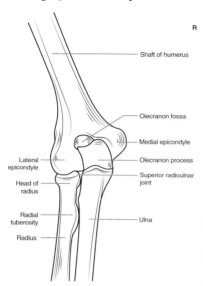

FIGURE 3.56   Anatomy of the AP projection of the right elbow.

Labels: R, Shaft of humerus, Olecranon fossa, Medial epicondyle, Lateral epicondyle, Olecranon process, Head of radius, Superior radioulnar joint, Radial tuberosity, Ulna, Radius

Resultant Image

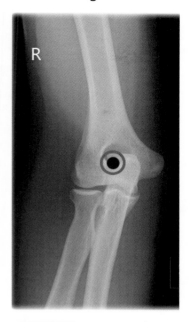

FIGURE 3.57   Resultant image of the AP projection of the right elbow.

Common positioning faults:

Additional projections:

Other notes:

Lateral Projection of the Elbow (Right)

Common Indications for Imaging

- Fracture of the olecranon process, radial head, distal humerus, e.g. supracondylar fracture
- Dislocation of the elbow
- Osteoarthritis

Radiographic Technique

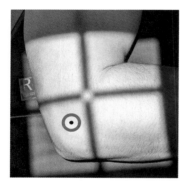

FIGURE 3.58 Patient positioning for the lateral elbow projection.

- Lower the shoulder to the same level as the forearm.
- Flex the elbow to 90° and rotate the forearm to the true lateral position with the thumb uppermost.
- Ensure that the medial aspect of the forearm is in contact with the IR.
- The medial and lateral epicondyles should be superimposed.
- Place the right anatomical marker in the primary beam – in this case on the right side of the right elbow.
- Collimate to include the proximal third of the forearm, the distal third of the humerus and the lateral borders of the elbow.

Centring point: with a vertical central ray at 90° to the IR to the lateral epicondyle of the right elbow.

Radiographic Anatomy

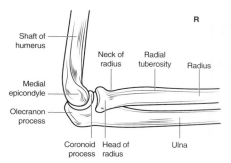

Shaft of humerus
Neck of radius
Radial tuberosity
Radius
R
Medial epicondyle
Olecranon process
Coronoid process
Head of radius
Ulna

FIGURE 3.59   Anatomy of the lateral elbow projection.

Resultant Image

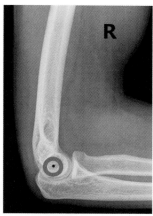

FIGURE 3.60   Resultant image of the lateral elbow projection.

Common positioning faults:

Additional projections:

Other notes:

Antero-posterior (AP) Projection of the Humerus (Left)

Common Indications for Imaging

- Fractures to humeral shaft
- Surgical neck fracture
- Supracondylar fracture

Radiographic Technique

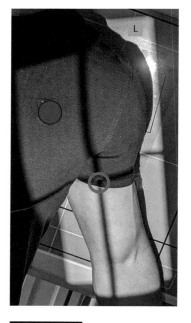

- Stand or sit the patient in front of the vertical IR facing the X-ray tube.
- Rotate the patient towards the affected side.
- Abduct the arm so that it is in the anatomical position and the posterior aspect of the shoulder, humerus and elbow are in contact with the IR.
- Place the left anatomical marker in the primary beam – in this case on the left side of the left humerus.
- Collimate to include the shoulder joint, elbow joint and the lateral borders of the humerus.

FIGURE 3.61 Patient positioning for the AP projection of the left humerus.

Centring point: with a horizontal central ray at 90° to the IR to the midshaft of the left humerus.

Radiographic Anatomy

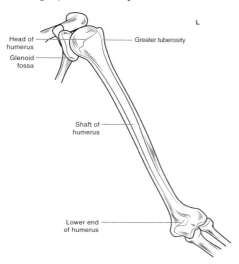

FIGURE 3.62 Anatomy of the AP projection of the left humerus.

Resultant Image

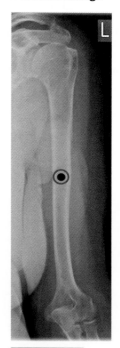

FIGURE 3.63 Resultant image of the AP projection of the left humerus.

Common positioning faults:	Other notes:
Additional projections:	

Lateral Projection of the Humerus (Left)

Common Indications for Imaging

- Fractures to humeral shaft
- Surgical neck fracture
- Supracondylar fracture

Radiographic Technique

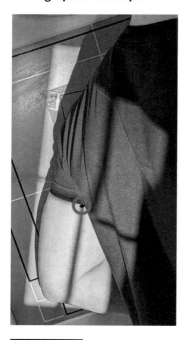

- Stand or sit the patient facing the vertical IR.
- Abduct and extend the arm and flex the elbow.
- Ensure that the lateral aspects of the shoulder, humerus and elbow are in contact with the IR.
- Place the left anatomical marker in the primary beam – in this case on the left side of the left humerus.
- Collimate to include the shoulder joint, elbow joint and the lateral borders of the humerus.

FIGURE 3.64   Patient positioning for the lateral humerus projection.

Centring point: with a horizontal central ray at 90° to the IR to the midshaft of the left humerus.

Radiographic Anatomy

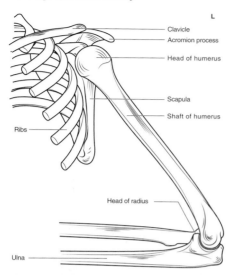

L

Clavicle
Acromion process
Head of humerus

Scapula
Shaft of humerus

Ribs

Head of radius

Ulna

FIGURE 3.65 Anatomy of the lateral humerus projection.

Resultant Image

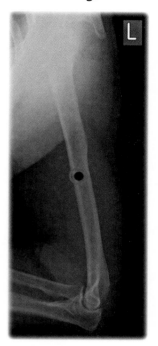

FIGURE 3.66 Resultant image of the lateral humerus projection.

Common positioning faults:

Additional projections:

Other notes:

CHAPTER **4**

Shoulder Girdle

This chapter will cover all the routine radiographic projections undertaken of the shoulder girdle. This will include the following projections.

- Shoulder
  - Antero-posterior (AP) Projection of the Shoulder (Right)
  - Supero-inferior (Axial) Projection of the Shoulder (Right)
- Scapula
  - Antero-posterior (AP) Projection of the Scapula (Right)
  - Lateral (Y) Projection of the Scapula (Right)
- Clavicle
  - Antero-posterior (AP) Projection of the Clavicle (Right)
  - Infero-superior Projection of the Clavicle (Right)

Fundamentals of Radiographic Positioning and Anatomy, First Edition.
Jane M. Harvey-Lloyd, Ruth M. Strudwick and Scott J. Preston.
© 2025 John Wiley & Sons Ltd. Published 2025 by John Wiley & Sons Ltd.

Antero-posterior (AP) Projection of the Shoulder (Right)

Common Indications for Imaging

- Osteoarthritis
- Fractures of the middle and outer third of the clavicle
- Fractures to the body, neck, acromion and coracoid processes of the scapula
- Dislocation of the shoulder joint – anterior or posterior
- Calcification of tendons
- Subluxation of the acromioclavicular joint
- Post shoulder joint replacement surgery

Radiographic Technique

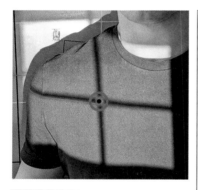

FIGURE 4.1 Patient positioning for the AP projection of the right shoulder.

- Stand the patient in the anatomical position, with the posterior aspect of the shoulder in contact with the IR.
- Rotate the patient 25° towards the affected side to allow visualisation of the glenohumeral joint.
- Turn the patient's head away from the affected side.
- Place the right anatomical marker in the primary beam – in this case on the right side of the right shoulder.
- Collimate to include from the superior skin borders of the shoulder to the inferior angle of the scapula, including the acromioclavicular joint and the sternoclavicular joint.

Centring Point: with a vertical central ray at 90° to the IR to the coracoid process of the right scapula.

Radiographic Anatomy

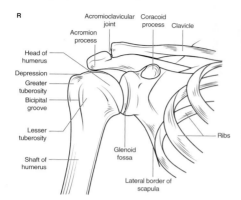

FIGURE 4.2   Anatomy of the AP projection of the right shoulder.

Resultant Image

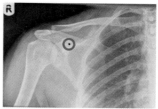

FIGURE 4.3   Resultant image of the AP projection of the right shoulder.

Common positioning faults:
Additional projections:

Other notes:

Supero-inferior (Axial) Projection of the Shoulder (Right)

Common Indications for Imaging

- Osteoarthritis
- Calcification of tendons
- Post shoulder joint replacement surgery

Radiographic Technique

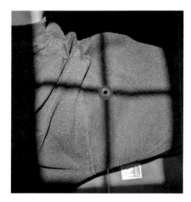

FIGURE 4.4 Patient positioning for the supero-inferior (axial) projection of the right shoulder.

- Seat the patient with the affected side nearest the IR.
- Adduct the patient's arm, flex the elbow and rest the forearm and hand on the IR so that palmar aspect of the hand is in contact with the IR. The patient should be leaning over the IR thus extending their shoulder joint as much as they are comfortable in doing so.
- Turn the patient's head away from the affected side.
- Place the right anatomical marker in the primary beam – in this case on the right side of the right shoulder.
- Collimate to include the skin borders laterally and the proximal third of the humerus and the glenoid cavity.

Centring Point: with a vertical central ray at 90° to the IR to the superior aspect of the head of humerus.

Radiographic Anatomy

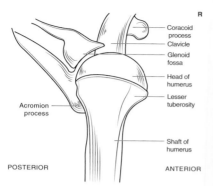

R
Coracoid process
Clavicle
Glenoid fossa
Head of humerus
Lesser tuberosity
Acromion process
Shaft of humerus
POSTERIOR
ANTERIOR

FIGURE 4.5 Anatomy of the supero-inferior (axial) projection of the right shoulder.

Resultant Image

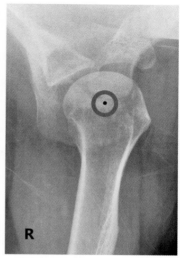

R

FIGURE 4.6 Resultant image of the supero-inferior (axial) projection of the right shoulder.

Common positioning faults:

Additional projections:

Other notes:

Antero-posterior (AP) Projection of the Scapula (Right)

Common Indications for Imaging

- Fractures to the body and neck of the scapula
- Fractures to acromion and coracoid processes of the scapula

Radiographic Technique

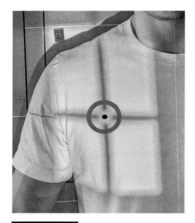

FIGURE 4.7 Patient positioning for the AP projection of the right scapula.

- Stand the patient in the anatomical position, with the posterior aspect of the shoulder in contact with the IR.
- Rotate the patient towards the affected side until the scapula is parallel to the IR.
- Turn the patient's head away from the affected side.
- Place the anatomical marker in the primary beam – in this case on the right side of the right shoulder.
- Collimate to include from the superior skin borders of the shoulder to the inferior angle of the scapula, including the acromioclavicular joint and the sternoclavicular joint.

Centring Point: with a vertical central ray at 90° to the IR to a point 2.5 cm below the midline of the right clavicle.

Radiographic Anatomy

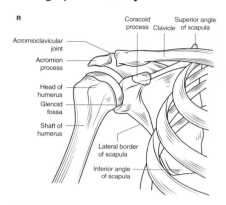

R

Coracoid
process Clavicle

Superior angle
of scapula

Acromioclavicular
joint

Acromion
process

Head of
humerus

Glenoid
fossa

Shaft of
humerus

Lateral border
of scapula

Inferior angle
of scapula

FIGURE 4.8 Anatomy of the AP projection of the right scapula.

Resultant Image

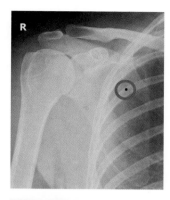

R

FIGURE 4.9 Resultant image of the AP projection of the right scapula.

Common positioning faults:

Additional projections:

Other notes:

Lateral (Y) Projection of the Scapula (Right)

Common Indications for Imaging

- Fractures to the body and neck of the scapula
- Fractures to acromion and coracoid processes of the scapula
- Dislocation of the shoulder joint

Radiographic Technique

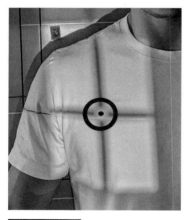

FIGURE 4.10 Patient positioning for the lateral (Y) projection of the right scapula.

- Stand the patient facing the IR.
- Rotate the patient so that the blade of the scapula is at 90° to the IR.
- Slightly adduct and extend the humerus and flex the elbow.
- Place the right anatomical marker in the primary beam – in this case on the right side of the right scapula.
- Collimate to include superior skin border of the shoulder, the glenoid cavity, the inferior angle of the scapula, the proximal third of the humerus and clavicle.

Centring Point: with a vertical central ray at 90° to the IR to the head of the humerus through the medial border of the right scapula and the level of T4.

Radiographic Anatomy

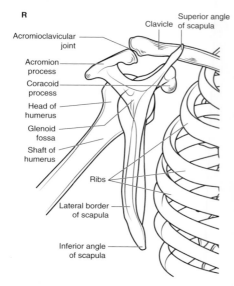

FIGURE 4.11   Anatomy of the lateral (Y) projection of the right scapula.

Resultant Image

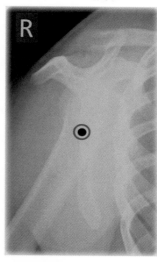

FIGURE 4.12   Resultant image of the lateral (Y) projection of the right scapula.

Common positioning faults:
Additional projections:

Other notes:

Antero-posterior (AP) Projection of the Clavicle (Right)

Common Indications for Imaging

- Fracture of the middle and outer thirds of the clavicle
- Subluxation of the acromioclavicular joint

Radiographic Technique

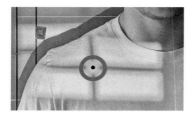

FIGURE 4.13 Patient positioning for the AP projection of the right clavicle.

- Stand the patient in the anatomical position, with the posterior aspect of the shoulder in contact with the IR.
- The patent should extend their elbow and let their arm rest at the side of their body.
- Turn the patient's head away from the affected side.
- Place the right anatomical marker in the primary beam – in this case on the right side of the right clavicle.
- Collimate to include the complete length of the clavicle.

Centring Point: with a vertical central ray at 90° to the IR to a point midway between the acromioclavicular and sternoclavicular joints on the right side.

Radiographic Anatomy

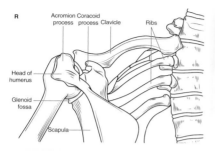

R

Acromion Coracoid
process process Clavicle   Ribs

Head of
humerus

Glenoid
fossa

Scapula

FIGURE 4.14   Anatomy of AP
projection of the right clavicle.

Resultant Image

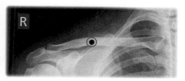

R

FIGURE 4.15   Resultant
image of the AP projection of the
right clavicle.

Common positioning faults:

Additional projections:

Other notes:

Infero-superior Projection of the Clavicle (Right)

Common Indications for Imaging

- Fracture of the middle and outer thirds of the clavicle
- Subluxation of the acromioclavicular joint

Radiographic Technique

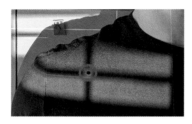

FIGURE 4.16   Patient positioning for the infero-superior projection of the right clavicle.

- Stand the patient in the anatomical position, with the posterior aspect of the shoulder in contact with the IR.
- The patent should extend their elbow and let their arm rest at the side of their body.
- Turn the patient's head away from the affected side.
- Place the right anatomical marker in the primary beam – in this case on the right side of the right clavicle.
- Collimate to include the complete length of the clavicle.

Centring Point: with a vertical central ray angled 30° cranially to a point midway between the acromioclavicular and sternoclavicular joints on the right side.

Radiographic Anatomy

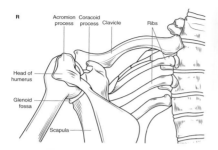

FIGURE 4.17   Anatomy of the infero-superior projection of the right clavicle.

Resultant Image

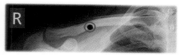

FIGURE 4.18   Resultant image of the infero-superior projection of the right clavicle.

Common positioning faults:

Additional projections:

Other notes:

CHAPTER 5

Lower Limb

This chapter will cover all the routine radiographic projections under-taken of the lower limb. This will include the following projections.

- Hallux
  - Dorsi-plantar (DP) Projection of the Hallux (Left)
  - Lateral Projection of Hallux (Left)
- Foot
  - Dorsi-plantar (DP) Projection of the Foot (Left)
  - Dorsi-plantar (DP) Oblique Projection of the Foot (Left)
  - Turned Lateral Projection of the Foot (Left)
- Calcaneum
  - Axial Projection of the Calcaneum (Left)
  - Lateral Projection of the Calcaneum (Left)
- Ankle
  - Antero-posterior (AP) Mortise Projection of the Ankle (Right)
  - Lateral Projection of the Ankle (Right)
- Tibia and Fibula
  - Antero-posterior (AP) Projection of the Tibia and Fibula (Tib/ Fib) (Left)
  - Lateral Projection of the Tibia and Fibula (Tib/ Fib) (Left)
- Knee
  - Antero-posterior Projection of the Knee (Left)
  - Turned Lateral Projection of the Knee (Left)
  - Horizontal Beam Lateral (HBL) Projection of the Knee (Right)
- Femur
  - Antero-posterior (AP) Projection of the Femur (Right) – Hip Down
  - Antero-posterior (AP) Projection of the Femur (Right) – Knee Up
  - Lateral Projection of the Femur (Right) – Hip Down
  - Lateral Projection of the Femur (Right) – Knee Up

Fundamentals of Radiographic Positioning and Anatomy, First Edition.
Jane M. Harvey-Lloyd, Ruth M. Strudwick and Scott J. Preston.
© 2025 John Wiley & Sons Ltd. Published 2025 by John Wiley & Sons Ltd.

Dorsi-plantar (DP) Projection of the Hallux (Left)

Common Indications for Imaging

- Fractures of base of first metatarsal
- Fractures of phalanges
- Dislocation of interphalangeal or metatarsophalangeal joint
- Osteoarthritis
- Hallux valgus

Radiographic Technique

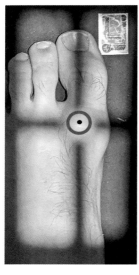

- Seat the patient with the hips and knee flexed and the foot in contact with the IR.
- Encourage the patient to relax their toes and ensure the toes are not flexed.
- Place the left anatomical marker in the primary beam – in this case on the left side of the great toe.
- Collimate to include superiorly the distal phalanx, inferiorly the metatarsophalangeal joint and laterally the soft tissue borders.

FIGURE 5.1   Patient positioning for the DP projection of the left hallux.

Centring point: with a vertical central ray at 90° to the IR at the first metatarsophalangeal joint of the left great toe.

Radiographic Anatomy

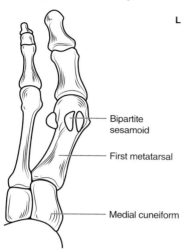

Bipartite sesamoid

First metatarsal

Medial cuneiform

FIGURE 5.2 Anatomy of the DP projection of the left hallux.

Resultant Image

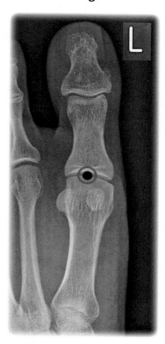

FIGURE 5.3 Resultant image of the DP projection of the left hallux.

Common positioning faults:
Additional projections:

Other notes:

Lateral Projection of Hallux (Left)

Common Indications for Imaging

- Fractures of base of first metatarsal
- Fractures of phalanges
- Dislocation of interphalangeal or metatarsal joint
- Osteoarthritis
- Hallux valgus

Radiographic Technique

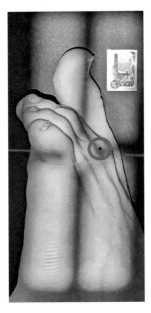

FIGURE 5.4 Patient positioning for lateral projection of the left hallux.

- Seat the patient with the leg extended on the affected side with the medial aspect of the hallux against the IR.
- Using a bandage, loop it around the other four toes and move them anteriorly or posteriorly, to allow for a lateral projection of the great toe to be acquired.
- This is a difficult position for the patient to remain in and therefore sometimes an oblique projection is adequate for diagnostic purposes.
- Place the left anatomical marker in the primary beam – in this case on the left side of the great toe.
- Collimate to include superiorly, the distal phalanx, inferiorly, the metatarsophalangeal joint and laterally the soft tissue borders.

Centring point: with a vertical central ray at 90° to the IR to the metatarsophalangeal joint of the left great toe.

Radiographic Anatomy

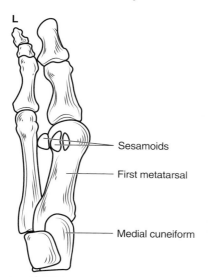

Sesamoids

First metatarsal

Medial cuneiform

FIGURE 5.5   Anatomy of the lateral projection of the left hallux.

Resultant Image

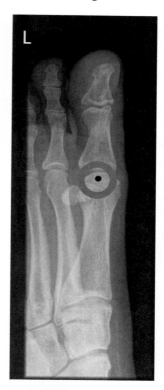

FIGURE 5.6   Resultant image of the lateral projection of the left hallux.

Common positioning faults:
Additional projections:

Other notes:

Dorsi-plantar (DP) Projection of the Foot (Left)

Common Indications for Imaging

- Fractures of tarsal or metatarsal bones
- Fractures of phalanges
- Dislocations
- Foreign body
- Osteoarthritis

Radiographic Technique

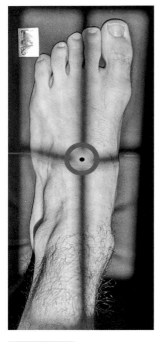

- Seat the patient on the examination table, with the knee on the affected side flexed.
- Place the plantar aspect of the foot flat on the IR.
- Place the left anatomical marker in the primary beam – in this case on the left side of the left foot.
- Can also be performed weight bearing with the patient gently standing on the image receptor or a protective, radiolucent cover.
- Consider application of a cranial angle on the X-ray tube of 8° to account for the arch of the foot.
- Collimate to include superiorly the distal phalanges, inferiorly the tarsal bones and laterally the soft tissue borders.

FIGURE 5.7 Patient positioning for DP projection of the left foot.

Centring point: with a vertical central ray at 90° at the cuboid-navicular joint of the left foot.

Radiographic Anatomy

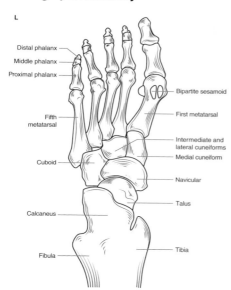

L

Distal phalanx
Middle phalanx
Proximal phalanx

Fifth
metatarsal

Cuboid

Calcaneus

Fibula

Bipartite sesamoid

First metatarsal

Intermediate and
lateral cuneiforms
Medial cuneiform

Navicular

Talus

Tibia

FIGURE 5.8   Anatomy of the DP projection of the left foot.

Resultant Image

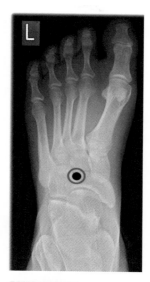

FIGURE 5.9   Resultant image of the DP projection of the left foot.

Common positioning faults:

Additional projections:

Other notes:

Dorsi-plantar (DP) Oblique Projection of the Foot (Left)

Common Indications for Imaging

- Fractures of base of metatarsals and phalanges
- Osteoarthritis
- Rheumatoid arthritis
- Lisfranc fracture
- Foreign body

Radiographic Technique

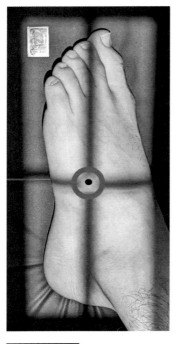

- Seat the patient on the examination table with the knee of the affected side flexed.
- Place the plantar aspect of the affected foot on the IR.
- Place a foam pad or ask the patient to medially rotate the leg to lift the lateral border of the foot to an angle of around 30–40°.
- Place the left anatomical marker in the primary beam – in this case on the left side of the left foot.
- Collimate to include superiorly the distal phalanges, inferiorly the calcaneum and laterally the soft tissue borders.

FIGURE 5.10 Patient positioning for the DP oblique projection of the left foot.

Centring point: with a vertical central ray at 90° to the IR at the cuboid-navicular joint of the left foot.

Radiographic Anatomy

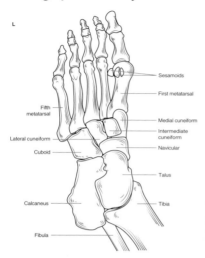

L

Sesamoids

First metatarsal

Fifth metatarsal

Medial cuneiform

Intermediate cuneiform

Lateral cuneiform

Navicular

Cuboid

Talus

Calcaneus

Tibia

Fibula

FIGURE 5.11   Anatomy of the DP oblique projection of the left foot.

Resultant Image

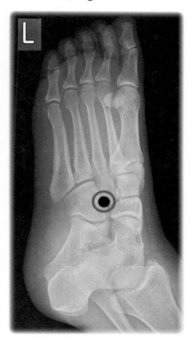

FIGURE 5.12   Resultant image of the DP oblique projection of the left foot.

Common positioning faults:
Additional projections:

Other notes:

Turned Lateral Projection of the Foot (Left)

Common Indications for Imaging

- Fractures of metatarsals, tarsals and phalanges
- Osteomyelitis
- Foreign body

Radiographic Technique

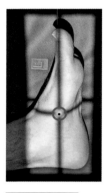

FIGURE 5.13   Patient positioning for the turned lateral projection of the left foot.

- Seat the patient on the examination table with the leg of the affected side externally rotated so the lateral aspect of the foot is in contact with the IR and the plantar aspect of the foot perpendicular to the IR.
- Have the patient apply a slight dorsiflexion.
- Place the left anatomical marker in the primary beam – in this case on the left side, superior to the dorsal aspect of the left foot.
- Collimate to include superiorly and inferiorly the soft tissue borders and laterally the distal phalanges and calcaneum.

Centring point: with a vertical central ray at 90° to the IR at the approximate level of the navicular of the left foot.

Radiographic Anatomy

L

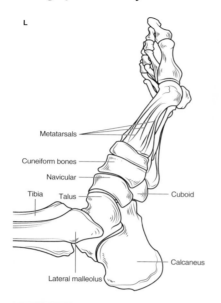

Metatarsals

Cuneiform bones

Navicular

Tibia   Talus

Cuboid

Calcaneus

Lateral malleolus

FIGURE 5.14 Anatomy of the turned lateral projection of the left foot.

Resultant Image

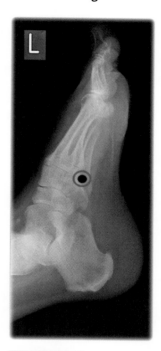

FIGURE 5.15 Resultant image of the turned lateral projection of the left foot.

Common positioning faults:

Additional projections:

Other notes:

Axial Projection of the Calcaneum (Left)

Common Indications for Imaging

- Fall from height landing directly on the calcaneal region (heel)
- Stress fracture of the calcaneum
- Foreign body

Radiographic Technique

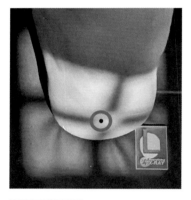

FIGURE 5.16 Patient positioning for the axial projection of the left calcaneum.

- Seat the patient on the examination table with the affected leg extended and the posterior aspect of the calcaneum (calcaneal tuberosity) on the IR.
- Using an apron or bandage or if the patient can manage without, apply dorsiflexion to the ankle.
- Place the left anatomical marker in the primary beam – in this case on the left side of the left calcaneum.
- Collimate to include superiorly and inferiorly the whole of the calcaneum and laterally the soft tissue borders.

Centring point: with a caudally angled X-ray tube at between 30° and 40° at the midplantar aspect of the left foot.

Radiographic Anatomy

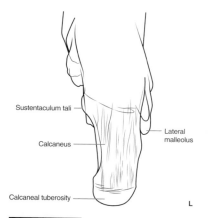

Sustentaculum tali

Calcaneus

Lateral malleolus

Calcaneal tuberosity

L

FIGURE 5.17   Anatomy of the axial projection of the left calcaneum.

Resultant Image

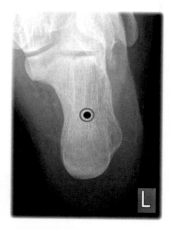

FIGURE 5.18   Resultant image of axial projection of the left calcaneum.

Common positioning faults:

Additional projections:

Other notes:

Lateral Projection of the Calcaneum (Left)

Common Indications for Imaging

- Fall from height directly on the calcaneal region (heel)
- Foreign body
- Stress fracture of the calcaneum

Radiographic Technique

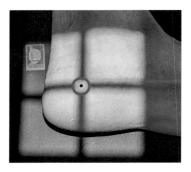

FIGURE 5.19 Patient positioning for the lateral projection of the left calcaneum.

- Lie the patient on the affected side.
- Extend the affected leg fully.
- Ensure the medial and lateral malleoli will be superimposed when projected.
- Place the left anatomical marker in the primary beam – in this case on the left side superior to the dorsum of the left foot.
- Collimate to include superiorly and inferiorly the soft tissue borders and laterally the whole of the calcaneal articulations.

Centring point: with a vertical central ray at 90° to the IR centred at the level of the taleo-calcaneal articulation of the left foot.

Radiographic Anatomy

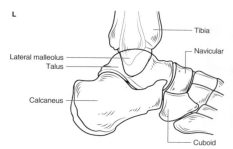

L

Tibia

Navicular

Lateral malleolus

Talus

Calcaneus

Cuboid

FIGURE 5.20 Anatomy of the lateral projection of the left calcaneum.

Resultant Image

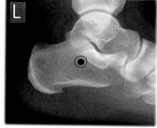

L

FIGURE 5.21 Resultant image of the lateral projection of the left calcaneum.

Common positioning faults:

Additional projections:

Other notes:

Antero-posterior (AP) Mortise Projection of the Ankle (Right)

Common Indications for Imaging

- Fracture of the ankle
- Fracture of base of fifth metatarsal
- Osteoarthritis

Radiographic Technique

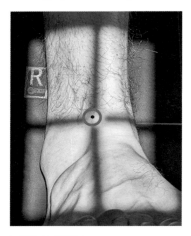

FIGURE 5.22 Patient positioning for the AP mortise projection of the right ankle.

- Sit or lie the patient with the legs extended.
- Abduct the unaffected leg.
- Place the heel of the foot on the IR with the joint flexed at 90°.
- Dorsiflex the foot.
- Rotate the ankle medially until the malleoli are equidistant from the IR.
- Place the right anatomical marker in the primary beam – in this case on the right side of the right ankle.
- Collimate to include superiorly, the distal third of the tibia and fibula, inferiorly, the midfoot and laterally, the soft tissue borders.

Centring point: with a vertical central ray at 90° to the IR centred midway between the malleoli of the right ankle.

Radiographic Anatomy

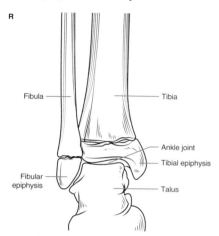

FIGURE 5.23   Anatomy of the AP mortise projection of the right ankle.

Resultant Image

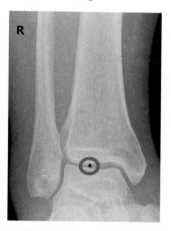

FIGURE 5.24   Resultant image of the AP mortise projection of the right Ankle.

Common positioning faults:
Additional projections:

Other notes:

Lateral Projection of the Ankle (Right)

Common Indications for Imaging

- Fracture of the ankle
- Fracture of base of fifth metatarsal
- Osteoarthritis

Radiographic Technique

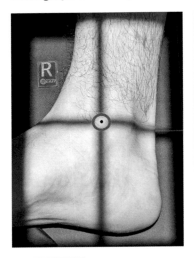

FIGURE 5.25 Patient positioning for the lateral projection of the right ankle.

- Lie the patient on the affected side.
- Extend the affected leg fully.
- Ensure the medial and lateral malleoli will be superimposed when projected.
- The tibia should be parallel to the IR.
- Place the right anatomical marker in the primary beam – in this case on the right side of the right ankle.
- Collimate to include superiorly the distal third of the tibia and fibula, inferiorly the base of the fifth metatarsal and laterally the soft tissue borders.

Centring point: with a vertical central ray at 90° to the IR centred at the medial malleolus of the right ankle.

Radiographic Anatomy

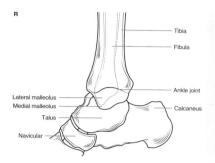

R

- Tibia
- Fibula
- Ankle joint
- Lateral malleolus
- Medial malleolus
- Calcaneus
- Talus
- Navicular

FIGURE 5.26   Anatomy of the lateral projection of the right ankle.

Resultant Image

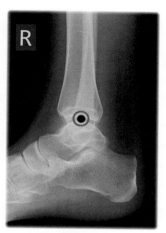

FIGURE 5.27   Resultant image of the lateral projection of the right ankle.

Common positioning faults:

Additional projections:

Other notes:

Antero-posterior (AP) Projection of the Tibia and Fibula (Tib/Fib) (Left)

Common Indications for Imaging

- Fracture of the tibia or fibula
- Foreign body
- Suspected malignancies
- Postoperative imaging (e.g. tibial intermedullary nail)

Radiographic Technique

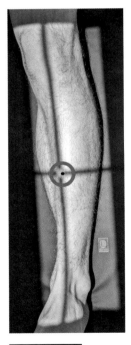

FIGURE 5.28 Patient positioning for the AP projection of the left tibia and fibula.

- Lie the patient on the examination table with the affected leg extended.
- Abduct the unaffected leg.
- Ensure the knee and ankle are in the AP position. N.B. Not an ankle mortise as this will displace the patella.
- You may need to rotate the IR so that the length from corner to corner can be used.
- It may be necessary to undertake dedicated projections of the knee and/or ankle joint.
- Place the left anatomical marker in the primary beam – in this case on the left side of the left tibia and fibula.
- Collimate to include superiorly the knee joint, inferiorly the ankle joint and laterally the soft tissue borders.

Centring point: with the central ray at 90° to the IR, centre midway between the knee and ankle joints of the left leg.

Radiographic Anatomy

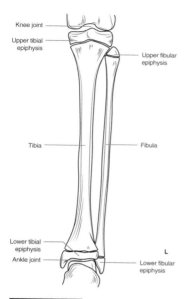

Knee joint

Upper tibial epiphysis

Upper fibular epiphysis

Tibia

Fibula

Lower tibial epiphysis

Ankle joint

L

Lower fibular epiphysis

FIGURE 5.29   Anatomy of the AP projection of the left tibia and fibula.

Resultant Image

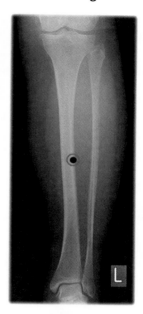

FIGURE 5.30   Resultant image of the AP projection of the left tibia and fibula.

Common positioning faults:	Other notes:
Additional projections:	

Lateral Projection of the Tibia and Fibula (Tib/Fib) (Left)

Common Indications for Imaging

- Malignancies
- Fracture of the tibia or fibula
- Foreign body
- Postoperative imaging (e.g. tibial intermedullary nail)

Radiographic Technique

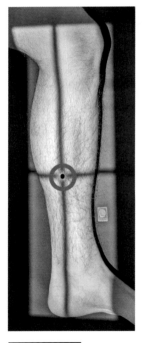

- With the patient lying on the affected side, flex the knee and hip as if undertaking a turned lateral knee projection and place the IR under the lower limb.

- Ensure the entire length of the tibia and fibula is on the IR.

- It may be necessary to undertake dedicated projections of the knee and/or ankle joint.

- Place the anatomical marker in the primary beam – in this case on the left side of the left tibia and fibula.

- Collimate to include superiorly the knee joint, inferiorly the ankle joint and laterally the soft tissue borders.

FIGURE 5.31 Patient positioning for the lateral projection of the left tibia and fibula.

Centring point: the central ray should be vertical and at 90° to the IR at the medial aspect of the lower limb approximately halfway between the knee and ankle joints of the left leg.

Radiographic Anatomy

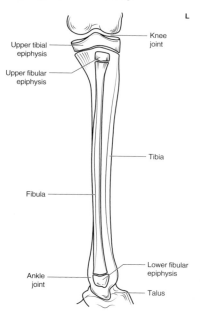

FIGURE 5.32   Anatomy of the lateral projection of the left tibia and fibula.

Resultant Image

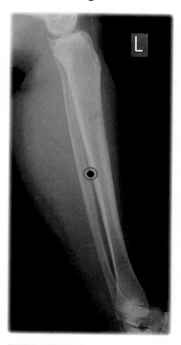

FIGURE 5.33   Resultant image of the lateral projection of the left tibia and fibula.

Common positioning faults:

Additional projections:

Other notes:

Antero-posterior Projection of the Knee (Left)

Common Indications for Imaging

- Fracture of the distal femur or proximal tibia/fibula
- Fracture of the patella
- Suspected abnormalities of the knee joint
- Osteoarthritis
- Foreign body

Radiographic Technique

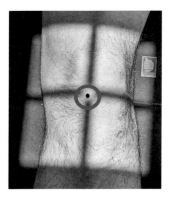

FIGURE 5.34 Patient positioning for the AP projection of the left knee.

- Lie the patient on the examination table with the legs extended and slightly abduct the unaffected leg.
- Internally rotate the leg to move the patella so that it is in the midline between the femoral condyles.
- Place the left anatomical marker in the primary beam – in this case on the left side of the left knee.
- This projection can also be carried out weight bearing.
- Collimate to include superiorly the distal third of the femur, inferiorly the proximal third of the tibia and fibula and laterally the soft tissue borders.

Centring point: the central ray should be vertical and at 90° to the IR approximately 2.5 cm below the apex of the patella of the left knee.

Radiographic Anatomy

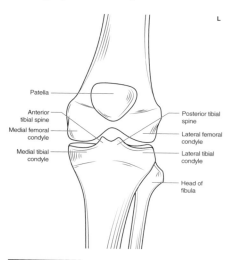

Patella

Anterior tibial spine

Medial femoral condyle

Medial tibial condyle

Posterior tibial spine

Lateral femoral condyle

Lateral tibial condyle

Head of fibula

FIGURE 5.35   Anatomy of the AP projection of the left knee.

Resultant Image

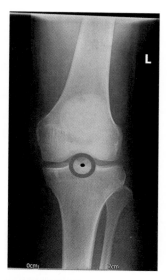

FIGURE 5.36   Resultant image of the AP projection of the left knee.

Common positioning faults:

Additional projections:

Other notes:

Turned Lateral Projection of the Knee (Left)

Common Indications for Imaging

- Fracture of the tibia, fibula or femur
- Fracture of the patella
- Suspected abnormalities of the knee joint
- Foreign body
- Osteoarthritis

Radiographic Technique

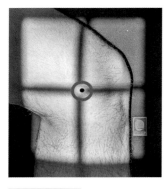

FIGURE 5.37 Patient positioning for the turned lateral projection of the left knee.

- Lie the patient on the affected side, flex the hip and knee.
- Place the lateral aspect of the knee joint against the IR.
- Aim for knee flexion of no more than 30°.
- The patella should be perpendicular to the IR with the tibia and fibula lying parallel to the IR.
- You may need to raise the ankle using a sandbag/wedge or rest it on the unaffected leg.
- Place the left anatomical marker in the primary beam – in this case on the left side of the left knee.
- Collimate to include superiorly the distal third of the femur, inferiorly the proximal third of the tibia and fibula and laterally the soft tissue borders.

Centring point: the central ray should be vertical and at 90° to the IR centred at a point 2.5 cm inferior and posterior to the apex of the patella of the left knee.

Radiographic Anatomy

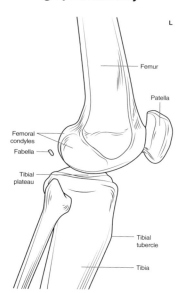

Femur

Patella

Femoral
condyles

Fabella

Tibial
plateau

Tibial
tubercle

Tibia

L

FIGURE 5.38   Anatomy of the
turned lateral projection of the
left knee.

Resultant Image

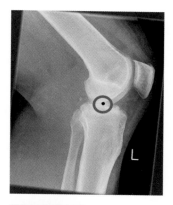

FIGURE 5.39   Resultant
image of the turned lateral
projection of the left knee.

Common positioning faults:

Additional projections:

Other notes:

Horizontal Beam Lateral (HBL) Projection of the Knee (Right)

Common Indications for Imaging

- Trauma
- Fracture of the tibia/fibula or femur
- Fracture of the patella

Radiographic Technique

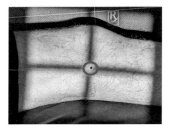

FIGURE 5.40   Patient positioning for the HBL knee projection.

- The patient should present lying down with the legs extended and the unaffected limb abducted slightly.
- Gently apply a pad under the knee joint for support and to raise it from the examination table or patient trolley (N.B. not an angled pad).
- Place the IR between the patient's legs and use a sand-bag or the patient to ensure it remains upright.
- Place the right anatomical marker in the primary beam – in this case superior to the anterior aspect on the right side of the right knee.
- Collimate to include superiorly the patella, inferiorly the soft tissue border and laterally the distal third of the femur and proximal third of the tibia and fibula.

Centring point: the central ray should be horizontal at 90° to the IR centred at a point 2.5 cm inferior and posterior to the apex of the patella of the left knee.

Radiographic Anatomy

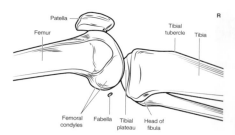

FIGURE 5.41   Anatomy of the HBL knee projection.

Resultant Image

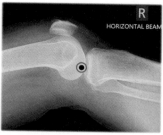

FIGURE 5.42   Resultant image of the HBL knee projection.

Common positioning faults:

Additional projections:

Other notes:

Antero-posterior (AP) Projection of the Femur (Right) – Hip Down

Common Indications for Imaging

- Fracture of the femur
- Suspected malignancy

Radiographic Technique

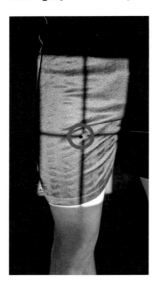

FIGURE 5.43 Patient positioning for the AP projection of the right femur – hip down.

- With the patient lying on the examination table, abduct the unaffected leg.
- Internally rotate the hip joint of the affected side to position the femur in the anatomical position with the patella superimposed over the distal femur.
- Aim to include the proximal 2/3 of the femur in this projection. If the whole femur is required, undertake an AP knee projection as well as this one.
- Place the right anatomical marker in the primary beam – in this case on the right side of the right knee.
- Collimate to include superiorly the hip joint, inferiorly the mid third of the femur and laterally the soft tissue borders.

Centring point: the central ray should be vertical and at 90° to the IR at the midpoint of the right femur.

Radiographic Anatomy

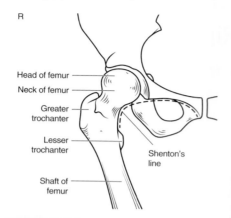

Head of femur
Neck of femur
Greater trochanter
Lesser trochanter
Shenton's line
Shaft of femur

R

FIGURE 5.44 Anatomy of the AP projection of the right femur – hip down.

Resultant Image

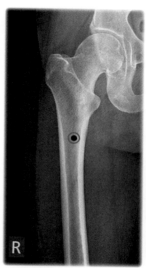

R

FIGURE 5.45 Resultant image of the AP projection of the right femur – hip down.

Common positioning faults:

Additional projections:

Other notes:

Antero-posterior (AP) Projection of the Femur (Right) – Knee Up

Common Indications for Imaging

- Fracture of the femur
- Suspected malignancy

Radiographic Technique

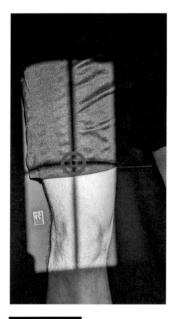

FIGURE 5.46 Patient positioning for the AP projection of the right femur – knee up.

- With the patient lying on the examination table, abduct the unaffected leg.
- Internally rotate the hip joint of the affected side to position the femur in the anatomical position with the patella superimposed over the distal femur.
- Place the right anatomical marker in the primary beam – in this case on the right side of the right knee.
- Aim to include the distal 2/3 of the femur in this projection. If the whole femur is required, undertake an AP hip projection as well as this one.
- Collimate to include superiorly at least the mid third of the femur, inferiorly the knee joint and laterally the soft tissue borders.

Centring point: the central ray should be vertical and at 90° to the IR at the midpoint of the right femur.

Radiographic Anatomy

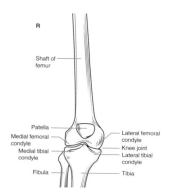

R

Shaft of
femur

Patella
Medial femoral
condyle
Medial tibial
condyle
Fibula

Lateral femoral
condyle
Knee joint
Lateral tibial
condyle
Tibia

FIGURE 5.47   Anatomy of
the AP projection of the right
femur – knee up.

Resultant Image

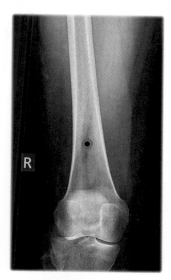

FIGURE 5.48   Resultant
image of the AP projection of
the right femur – knee up.

Common positioning faults:

Additional projections:

Other notes:

Lateral Projection of the Femur (Right) – Hip Down

Common Indications for Imaging

- Fracture
- Malignancy
- Foreign body

Radiographic Technique

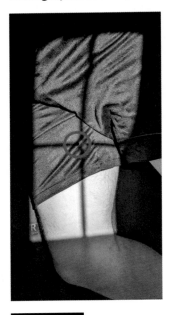

FIGURE 5.49 Patient positioning for the lateral projection of the right femur – hip down.

- With the patient lying on the affected side, place the lateral aspect of the affected limb against the IR.
- You may wish to place a pad under the ankle for support and comfort.
- Aim to include the proximal 2/3 of the femur in this projection. If a whole femur is required, undertake a lateral knee projection.
- In cases of significant trauma or where a fracture is noted on the AP projection, you may wish to raise the unaffected limb and utilise the upright bucky to undertake an HBL projection.
- Place the right anatomical marker in the primary beam.
- Collimate to include superiorly and inferiorly, the soft tissue border, and laterally the hip joint and mid third of the femur.

Centring point: the central ray should be vertical and at 90° to the IR centred at the medial midthigh area of the right leg.

Radiographic Anatomy

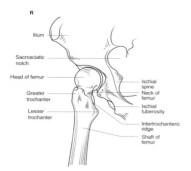

FIGURE 5.50 Anatomy of the lateral projection of the right femur – hip down.

Resultant Image

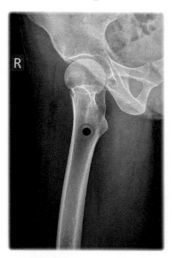

FIGURE 5.51 Resultant image of the lateral projection of the right femur – hip down.

Common positioning faults:	Other notes:
Additional projections:	

Lateral Projection of the Femur (Right) – Knee Up

Common Indications for Imaging

- Fracture
- Malignancy
- Foreign body

Radiographic Technique

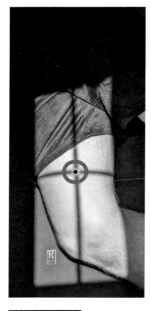

FIGURE 5.52 Patient positioning for the lateral projection of the right femur – knee up.

- With the patient lying on the affected side, place the lateral aspect of the affected limb against the IR.
- You may wish to place a pad under the ankle for support and comfort.
- Aim to include the distal 2/3 of the femur in this projection. If a whole femur is required, undertake a lateral hip projection.
- In cases of significant trauma or where a fracture is noted on the AP projection, you may wish to raise the unaffected limb and utilise the upright bucky to undertake an HBL projection.
- Place the right anatomical marker in the primary beam.
- Collimate to include superiorly and inferiorly the soft tissue border, and laterally the knee joint and mid third of the femur.

Centring point: the central ray should be vertical and at 90° to the IR centred at the medial midthigh area of the right leg.

Radiographic Anatomy

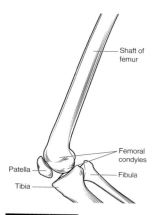

Shaft of
femur

Femoral
condyles

Patella

Fibula

Tibia

FIGURE 5.53   Anatomy of the
lateral projection of the right
femur – knee up.

Resultant Image

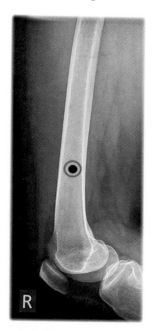

R

FIGURE 5.54   Resultant
image of the lateral
projection of the right
femur – knee up.

Common positioning faults:

Additional projections:

Other notes:

CHAPTER **6**

Pelvic Girdle

This chapter will cover all the routine radiographic projections under-taken of the pelvic girdle. This will include the following projections.

- Pelvis
  - Antero-Posterior (AP) Projection of the Pelvis
  - 'Low Centred' Antero-Posterior (AP) Projection of the Pelvis
- Hip Joint
  - Antero-Posterior (AP) Projection of the Hip Joint (Left)
  - Turned Lateral Projection of the Hip Joint (Left)
  - Horizontal-Beam Lateral Projection of the Hip Joint (Left)
- SacroIlliac Joints
  - Postero-Anterior (PA) Projection of the Sacroiliac Joints

Fundamentals of Radiographic Positioning and Anatomy, First Edition.
Jane M. Harvey-Lloyd, Ruth M. Strudwick and Scott J. Preston.
© 2025 John Wiley & Sons Ltd. Published 2025 by John Wiley & Sons Ltd.

Antero-posterior (AP) Projection of the Pelvis

Common Indications for Imaging

- Osteoarthritis
- Pelvic fractures
- Neck of femur fractures
- Hip dislocation
- Suspected bone tumour

Radiographic Technique

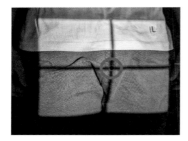

FIGURE 6.1 Patient positioning for the AP pelvis projection.

- Lie the patient supine on the table.
- Ensure that the median sagittal plane is parallel to the tabletop and perpendicular to the IR and the anterior superior iliac spines (ASIS) are equidistant from the IR.
- Ensure that the patient is not rotated.
- Rotate both legs medially, so that the toes are together and heels apart – if a fracture to the neck of femur is suspected, the legs should not be rotated.
- Place the anatomical marker in the primary beam on the correct anatomical side.
- Collimate to include the iliac crests superiorly, the proximal third of the femurs inferiorly and the skin borders laterally.

Centring point: with a vertical central ray at 90° to the IR in the midline 2.5 cm above the superior border of the symphysis pubis.

Radiographic Anatomy

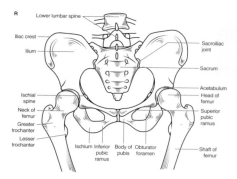

FIGURE 6.2 Anatomy of the AP pelvis projection.

Resultant Image

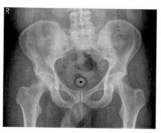

FIGURE 6.3 Resultant image of the AP pelvis projection.

Common positioning faults:

Additional projections:

Other notes:

'Low Centred' Antero-posterior (AP) Projection of the Pelvis

Common Indications for Imaging

- Preoperative assessment for total hip replacement or other hip joint surgery
- Postoperative assessment of total hip replacement or other hip joint surgery

Radiographic Technique

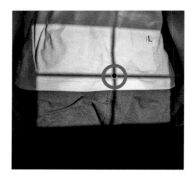

FIGURE 6.4 Patient positioning for the 'low centred' AP pelvis projection.

- Lie the patient supine on the table.
- Ensure that the median sagittal plane is parallel to the tabletop and perpendicular to the IR and the ASIS are equidistant from the IR.
- Ensure that the patient is not rotated.
- Rotate both legs medially, so that the toes are together and heels apart.
- Place the anatomical marker in the primary beam on the correct anatomical side.
- Collimate to include the ASIS superiorly, the proximal half of the femurs inferiorly and the skin borders laterally.

Centring point: with a vertical central ray at 90° to the IR in the midline at the superior border of the symphysis pubis.

Radiographic Anatomy

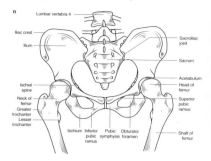

FIGURE 6.5 Anatomy for the 'low centred' AP pelvis projection.

Resultant Image

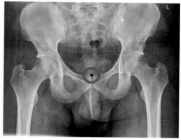

FIGURE 6.6 Resultant image of the 'low centred' AP pelvis projection.

Common positioning faults:

Additional projections:

Other notes:

Antero-posterior (AP) Projection of the Hip Joint (Left)

Common Indications for Imaging

- Assessment of unilateral hip pain
- Suspected unilateral hip pathology
- Assessment of unilateral hip pathology

Radiographic Technique

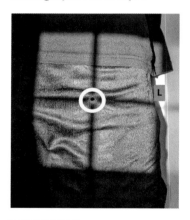

FIGURE 6.7 Patient positioning for the AP projection of the left hip joint.

- Lie the patient supine on the table.
- Ensure that the median sagittal plane is parallel to the tabletop and perpendicular to the IR.
- Ensure that the patient is not rotated with the ASIS are equidistant from the IR.
- Rotate both legs medially, so that the toes are together and heels apart – if a fracture to the neck of femur is suspected, the legs should not be rotated.
- Place the left anatomical marker in the primary beam on the left side of the left hip.
- Collimate to include the iliac crest superiorly, the proximal third of the femur inferiorly and the skin border laterally.

Centring point: with a vertical central ray at 90° to the IR over the hip joint at a point 2.5 cm distal along a perpendicular bisection of a line between the left anterior superior iliac spine and the superior border of the symphysis pubis.

Radiographic Anatomy

Resultant Image

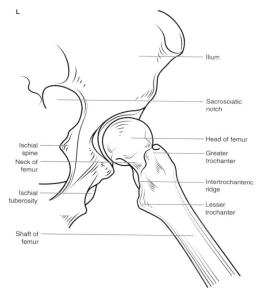

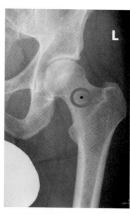

L

Ilium

Sacrosciatic notch

Head of femur

Ischial spine

Greater trochanter

Neck of femur

Intertrochanteric ridge

Ischial tuberosity

Lesser trochanter

Shaft of femur

FIGURE 6.9   Resultant image of the AP projection of the left hip joint.

FIGURE 6.8   Anatomy of for the AP projection of the left hip joint.

Common positioning faults:

Additional projections:

Other notes:

Turned Lateral Projection of the Hip Joint (Left)

Common Indications for Imaging

- Assessment of unilateral hip pain
- Suspected unilateral hip pathology
- Assessment of unilateral hip pathology

Radiographic Technique

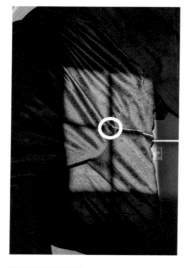

- Lie the patient on the affected side on the table with the hip and knee joints flexed.
- Ensure that the coronal plane and the pelvis are at 45° to the tabletop.
- Rest the unaffected leg in a comfortable position.
- Immobilise the patient.
- Place the left anatomical marker in the primary beam.
- Collimate to include the iliac crest superiorly, the proximal third of the femur inferiorly and the skin borders laterally.

FIGURE 6.10   Patient positioning for the turned lateral projection of the left hip joint.

Centring point: with a vertical central ray at 90° to the IR over the left hip joint.

Radiographic Anatomy

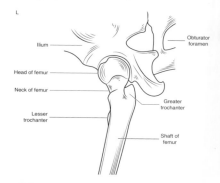

L

Ilium

Head of femur

Neck of femur

Lesser trochanter

Obturator foramen

Greater trochanter

Shaft of femur

FIGURE 6.11   Anatomy of the turned lateral projection of the left hip.

Resultant Image

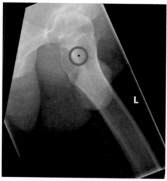

L

FIGURE 6.12   Resultant image of the turned lateral projection of the left hip.

Common positioning faults:

Additional projections:

Other notes:

Horizontal Beam Lateral Projection of the Hip Joint (Right)

Common Indications for Imaging

- Neck of femur fractures
- Total hip replacement
- Dislocation

Radiographic Technique

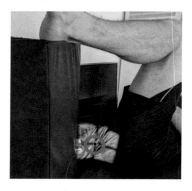

FIGURE 6.13 Patient positioning for the horizontal beam lateral projection of the right hip joint.

- Lie the patient supine on the table.
- Ensure that the median sagittal plane is parallel to the tabletop and perpendicular to the IR.
- Ensure that the patient is not rotated.
- Flex the unaffected hip and raise the unaffected leg, place the patient's foot on a support, and flex the unaffected knee to 90°.
- Place the left anatomical marker in the primary beam.
- Collimate to include the affected neck of femur and the skin borders superiorly and inferiorly.

Centring point: with a horizontal central ray at 90° to the IR over the left hip joint in the groin.

Radiographic Anatomy

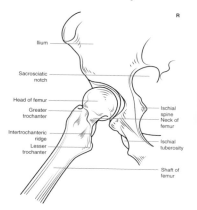

R

Ilium

Sacrosciatic
notch

Head of femur

Greater
trochanter

Intertrochanteric
ridge

Lesser
trochanter

Ischial
spine

Neck of
femur

Ischial
tuberosity

Shaft of
femur

FIGURE 6.14   Anatomy of the horizontal beam lateral projection of the right hip joint.

Resultant Image

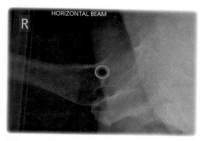

FIGURE 6.15   Resultant image of the horizontal beam lateral projection of the right hip joint.

Common positioning faults:

Additional projections:

Other notes:

Postero-anterior (PA) Projection of the Sacroiliac Joints

Common Indications for Imaging

- Suspected sacroiliitis
- Suspected ankylosing spondylitis

Radiographic Technique

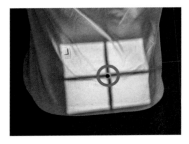

FIGURE 6.16 Patient positioning for the PA projection of the sacroiliac joints.

- Lie the patient prone on the table.
- Ensure that the median sagittal plane is parallel to the tabletop and perpendicular to the IR and the posterior anterior iliac spines (PSIS) are equidistant from the IR.
- Ensure that the patient is not rotated.
- Ask the patient to rest on their elbows.
- Place the anatomical marker in the primary beam.
- Collimate to include the sacroiliac joints with the iliac crests superiorly.

Centring point: with a vertical central ray at 90° to the IR in the midline at the level of the posterior superior iliac spines.

Radiographic Anatomy

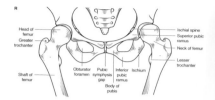

FIGURE 6.17   Anatomy of for the PA projection of the sacroiliac joints.

Resultant Image

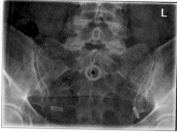

FIGURE 6.18   Resultant image of the PA projection of the sacroiliac joints.

Common positioning faults:

Additional projections:

Other notes:

CHAPTER 7

Spine

This chapter will cover all the routine radiographic projections undertaken of the spine. This will include the following projections.

- Cervical Spine
  - Antero-posterior (AP) Projection of the Cervical Spine
  - Lateral Projection of the Cervical Spine (Right)
  - Antero-posterior (AP) Open Mouth Odontoid Process (Peg) Projection
- Thoracic Spine
  - Antero-posterior (AP) Projection of the Thoracic Spine
  - Lateral Projection of the Thoracic Spine (Right)
- Lumbar Spine
  - Antero-posterior (AP) Projection of the Lumbar Spine
  - Lateral Projection of the Lumbar Spine (Right)

Fundamentals of Radiographic Positioning and Anatomy, First Edition.
Jane M. Harvey-Lloyd, Ruth M. Strudwick and Scott J. Preston.
© 2025 John Wiley & Sons Ltd. Published 2025 by John Wiley & Sons Ltd.

Antero-posterior (AP) Projection of the Cervical Spine

Common Indications for Imaging

- Osteoarthritis
- Cervical rib
- Schmorl's nodes
- Spondylolisthesis
- Fractures of the articular processes, spinous processes, transverse processes and vertebral bodies
- Dislocation

Radiographic Technique

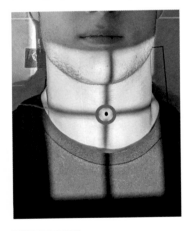

FIGURE 7.1 Patient positioning for the AP projection of the cervical spine.

- Stand the patient in the anatomical position, with the posterior aspect of the head and shoulders in contact with the IR.
- Check the head is not rotated by ensuring that the zygomas are equidistant from the IR.
- Raise the chin so that the symphysis menti will be superimposed over the occipital bone.
- Place the anatomical marker in the primary beam.
- Collimate to include from the base of the skull to the level of T1 and laterally to the skin borders.

Centring point: with a vertical central ray angle 15° cranially and centre to the midline 5 cm superior to the suprasternal notch.

Radiographic Anatomy

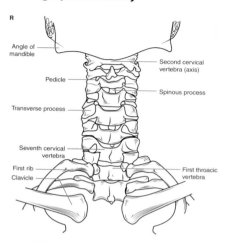

R

Angle of mandible

Pedicle

Transverse process

Seventh cervical vertebra

First rib

Clavicle

Second cervical vertebra (axis)

Spinous process

First throacic vertebra

FIGURE 7.2 Anatomy of the AP projection of the cervical spine.

Resultant Image

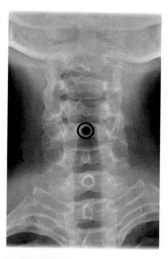

FIGURE 7.3 Resultant image of the AP projection of the cervical spine.

Common positioning faults:

Additional projections:

Other notes:

Lateral Projection of the Cervical Spine (Right)

Common Indications for Imaging

- Osteoarthritis
- Schmorl's nodes
- Spondylolisthesis
- Fractures of the articular processes, spinous processes, transverse processes and vertebral bodies
- Dislocation

Radiographic Technique

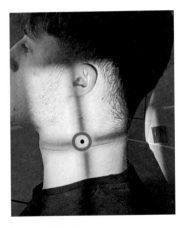

FIGURE 7.4 Patient positioning for right lateral projection of the cervical spine.

- Stand the patient in the true lateral position with the affected (right) side nearest the IR.
- Raise the patent's chin slightly so the angle of the mandible is clear of the cervical spine.
- Ask the patient to relax their shoulders or use weighted bags.
- Place the right anatomical marker in the primary beam.
- Collimate to include from the external auditory meatus superiorly to the level of T1 inferiorly and the soft tissue borders laterally.

Centring point: a source-to-image distance of at least 150 cm should be used with a horizontal central ray to a point 2.5 cm posterior to the angle of the left mandible, at the level of the thyroid cartilage.

Radiographic Anatomy

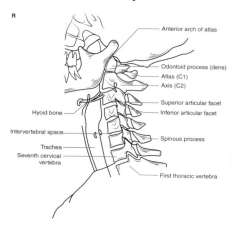

FIGURE 7.5   Anatomy of the lateral projection of the cervical spine.

Resultant Image

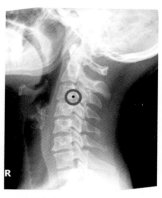

FIGURE 7.6   Resultant image of the lateral projection of the cervical spine.

Common positioning faults:

Additional projections:

Other notes:

Antero-posterior (AP) Open Mouth Odontoid Process (Peg) Projection

Common Indications for Imaging

- Fracture through the waist of the odontoid peg

Radiographic Technique

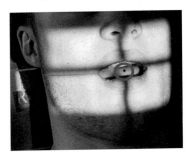

FIGURE 7.7 Patient positioning for the AP projection of the open mouth odontoid process (Peg) projection.

- Stand the patient in the anatomical position, with the posterior aspect of the head and shoulders in contact with the IR.
- Check the head is not rotated by ensuring that the zygomas are equidistant from the IR.
- Extend the patient's head so that the radiographic baseline is 20° from the horizontal.
- Ask the patient to open their mouth and recheck all the positioning.
- Place the anatomical marker in the primary beam.
- Collimate to include the base of skull superiorly, the level of C2 inferiorly and the lateral masses of C2 laterally.

Centring point: with a vertical central ray at 90° to the IR to the centre of the open mouth.

Radiographic Anatomy

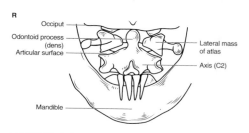

FIGURE 7.8   Anatomy of the AP open mouth odontoid process (Peg) projection.

Resultant Image

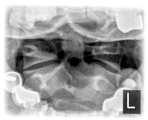

FIGURE 7.9   Resultant image of the AP projection of the open mouth odontoid process (Peg) projection.

Common positioning faults:
Additional projections:

Other notes:

Antero-posterior (AP) Projection of the Thoracic Spine

Common Indications for Imaging

- Osteoarthritis
- Schmorl's nodes
- Spondylolisthesis
- Fractures of the articular processes, spinous processes, transverse processes and vertebral bodies
- Scoliosis
- Osteoporosis
- Kyphosis

Radiographic Technique

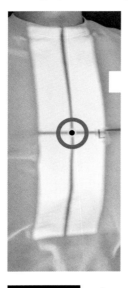

FIGURE 7.10 Patient positioning for the AP projection of the thoracic spine.

- Lie the patient supine, with the median sagittal plane perpendicular to the IR and the anterior superior iliac spines (ASIS) equidistant from the IR.
- Ask the patient to place their arms and hands by the side of their body.
- Place the anatomical marker in the primary beam.
- Collimate to include from the level of C7 superiorly to T12 inferiorly and the lateral borders of the vertebral bodies laterally.

Centring point: with a vertical central ray at 90° to the IR in the midline midway between the suprasternal notch and the xiphoid process.

Radiographic Anatomy

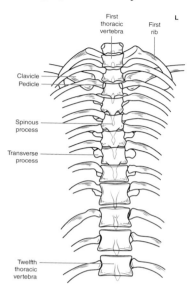

First thoracic vertebra

First rib

L

Clavicle
Pedicle

Spinous process

Transverse process

Twelfth thoracic vertebra

FIGURE 7.11   Anatomy of the AP projection of the thoracic spine.

Resultant Image

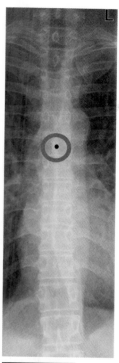

FIGURE 7.12   Resultant image of the AP projection of the thoracic spine.

Common positioning faults:

Additional projections:

Other notes:

Lateral Projection of the Thoracic Spine (Right)

Common Indications for Imaging

- Osteoarthritis
- Schmorl's nodes
- Spondylolisthesis
- Fractures of the articular processes, spinous processes, transverse processes and vertebral bodies
- Scoliosis
- Osteoporosis
- Kyphosis

Radiographic Technique

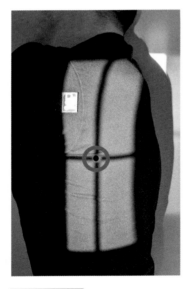

FIGURE 7.13 Patient positioning for the right lateral projection of the thoracic spine.

- Lie the patient in the true lateral position on their right side, with the median sagittal plane parallel to the IR.
- Ask the patient to raise their arms above their head and slightly flex their hips and knees for support.
- Ensure that the thoracic spine is parallel to the IR.
- Place the right anatomical marker in the primary beam.
- Collimate to include superiorly the level of T2–3 to T12 inferiorly and laterally to include the vertebral bodies and spinous processes.

Centring point: with a vertical central ray at 90° to the IR centre 5 cm anterior to the spinous process of T6.

Radiographic Anatomy

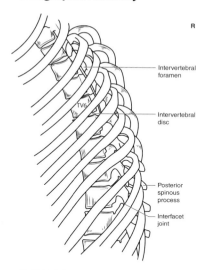

R

Intervertebral foramen

TV6

Intervertebral disc

Posterior spinous process

Interfacet joint

FIGURE 7.14   Anatomy of the right lateral projection of the thoracic spine.

Resultant Image

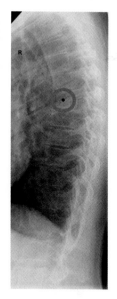

R

FIGURE 7.15   Resultant image of the right lateral projection of the thoracic spine.

Common positioning faults:

Additional projections:

Other notes:

Antero-posterior (AP) Projection of the Lumbar Spine

Common Indications for Imaging

- Osteoarthritis
- Schmorl's nodes
- Spondylolisthesis
- Fractures of the articular processes, spinous processes, transverse processes and vertebral bodies
- Scoliosis
- Lordosis
- Spina bifida
- Ankylosing spondylitis

Radiographic Technique

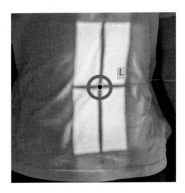

FIGURE 7.16 Patient positioning for the AP projection of the lumbar spine.

- Lie the patient supine, with the median sagittal plane perpendicular to the IR and the ASIS equidistant form the IR.
- Ask the patient to place their arms and hands by the side of their body.
- Allow the patient to flex their knees for comfort if needed.
- Place the anatomical marker in the primary beam.
- Collimate to include from the level of T12 superiorly to the sacroiliac joints inferiorly and laterally the lateral borders of the vertebral bodies to include the sacroiliac joints.

Centring point: with a vertical central ray at 90° to the IR in the midline at the level of L3.

Radiographic Anatomy

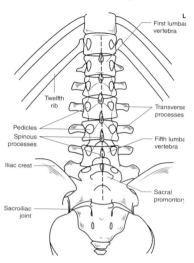

First lumbar
vertebra

Twelfth
rib

Transverse
processes

Pedicles
Spinous
processes

Fifth lumbar
vertebra

Iliac crest

Sacral
promontory

Sacroiliac
joint

FIGURE 7.17 Anatomy of the AP
projection of the lumbar spine.

Resultant Image

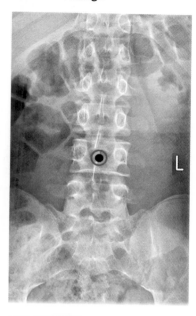

FIGURE 7.18 Resultant image of
the AP projection of the lumbar spine.

Common positioning faults:

Additional projections:

Other notes:

Lateral Projection of the Lumbar Spine (Right)

Common Indications for Imaging

- Osteoarthritis
- Schmorl's nodes
- Spondylolisthesis
- Fractures of the articular processes, spinous processes, transverse processes and vertebral bodies
- Scoliosis
- Lordosis
- Spina bifida
- Ankylosing spondylitis

Radiographic Technique

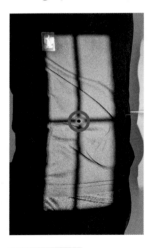

FIGURE 7.19   Patient positioning for the lateral lumbar spine projection.

- Lie the patient in the true lateral position, with the median sagittal plane parallel to the IR.
- Ask the patient to raise their arms above their head and slightly flex their hips and knees for support.
- Ensure that the lumbar spine is parallel to the IR, using pads if necessary.
- Place the right anatomical marker in the primary beam.
- Collimate to include from the level of L1 superiorly to the L5/SI joint inferiorly and laterally the vertebral bodies and spinous processes.

Centring point: with a vertical central ray at 90° to the IR centre 7.5 cm anterior to the spinous process of L3.

Radiographic Anatomy

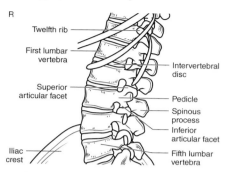

R

- Twelfth rib
- First lumbar vertebra
- Superior articular facet
- Iliac crest
- Intervertebral disc
- Pedicle
- Spinous process
- Inferior articular facet
- Fifth lumbar vertebra

FIGURE 7.20 Anatomy of the lateral lumbar spine projection.

Resultant Image

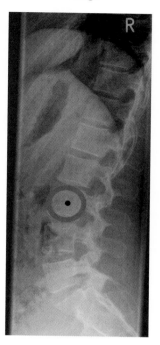

FIGURE 7.21 Resultant image of the lateral lumbar spine projection.

Common positioning faults:

Additional projections:

Other notes:

CHAPTER **8**

Skull and Facial Bones

This chapter will cover all the routine radiographic projections undertaken of the skull and facial bones. This will include the following projections.

- Skull
  - Occipito-Frontal (OF) 20° Projection of the Skull
  - Fronto-Occipital (FO) 30° (Towne's) Projection of the Skull
  - Lateral Projection of the Skull (Right)
- Facial Bones
  - Occipito-Mental (OM) Projection of the Facial Bones
  - Occipito-Mental (OM) 30° Projection of the Facial Bones
  - Lateral Projection of the Facial Bones (Right)
- Mandible
  - Postero-Anterior (PA) Projection of the Mandible
  - Lateral Oblique Projections of the Mandible (Right)
- Orbits
  - Occipito-Frontal (OF) 20° Projection of the Orbits
- Dental
  - Dental Panoramic Tomography (DPT)

Fundamentals of Radiographic Positioning and Anatomy, First Edition.
Jane M. Harvey-Lloyd, Ruth M. Strudwick and Scott J. Preston.
© 2025 John Wiley & Sons Ltd. Published 2025 by John Wiley & Sons Ltd.

Occipito-frontal (OF) 20° Projection of the Skull

Common Indications for Imaging

- Skull fractures
- Suspected bone tumour
- Location of foreign body

Radiographic Technique

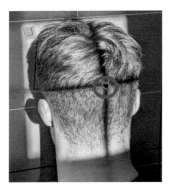

FIGURE 8.1 Patient positioning for the OF 20° skull projection.

- Sit the patient erect in a chair.
- Rest the patient's forehead and nose against the IR.
- Ensure that the radiographic baseline is parallel to the floor.
- Ensure that the interpupillary line is parallel to the floor.
- Ensure that the median sagittal plane is perpendicular to the IR.
- Ensure that the patient is not rotated.
- Place the anatomical marker in the primary beam.
- Collimate to include the skin borders.

Centring point: with a horizontal central ray angled 20° caudally in the midline with the beam exiting at the nasion.

Radiographic Anatomy

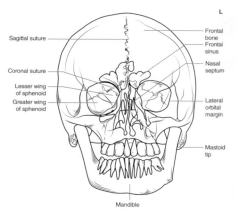

Sagittal suture
Coronal suture
Lesser wing of sphenoid
Greater wing of sphenoid

Frontal bone
Frontal sinus
Nasal septum
Lateral orbital margin
Mastoid tip

Mandible

FIGURE 8.2   Anatomy of the OF 20° skull projection.

Resultant Image

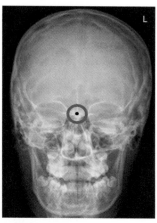

L

FIGURE 8.3   Resultant image of the OF 20° skull projection.

Common positioning faults:

Additional projections:

Other notes:

Fronto-occiptal (FO) 30° (Towne's) Projection of the Skull

Common Indications for Imaging

- Skull fractures
- Suspected bone tumour
- Location of foreign body

Radiographic Technique

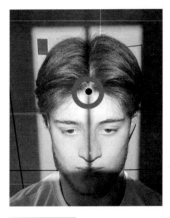

FIGURE 8.4 Patient positioning for the FO 30° (Towne's) projection of the skull.

- Sit the patient erect in a chair.
- Rest the back of the patient's head against the IR.
- Ensure that the radiographic baseline is parallel to the floor.
- Ensure that the interpupillary line is parallel to the floor.
- Ensure that the median sagittal plane is perpendicular to the IR.
- Ensure that the patient is not rotated.
- Place the anatomical marker in the primary beam.
- Collimate to include the skin borders.

Centring point: with a horizontal central ray angled 30° caudally in the midline 5 cm above the glabella.

Radiographic Anatomy

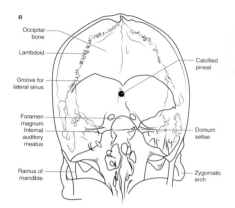

R
- Occipital bone
- Lambdoid
- Groove for lateral sinus
- Foramen magnum
- Internal auditory meatus
- Ramus of mandible
- Calcified pineal
- Dorsum sellae
- Zygomatic arch

FIGURE 8.5   Anatomy of the FO 30° (Towne's) projection of the skull.

Resultant Image

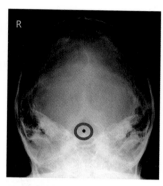

R

FIGURE 8.6   Resultant image of for the FO 30° (Towne's) projection of the skull.

Common positioning faults:

Additional projections:

Other notes:

Lateral Projection of the Skull (Right)

Common Indications for Imaging

- Skull fractures
- Suspected bone tumour
- Location of foreign body
- To check position of ventriculoperitoneal (VP) shunts

Radiographic Technique

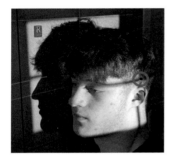

FIGURE 8.7 Patient positioning for the right lateral projection of the skull.

- Sit the patient erect in a chair.
- Turn the patient so that the right side of their head is in contact with the IR.
- Ensure that the radiographic baseline is parallel to the floor.
- Ensure that the interpupillary line is parallel to the floor.
- Ensure that the median sagittal plane is parallel to the IR.
- Ensure that the patient is not rotated.
- Place the right anatomical marker in the primary beam.
- Collimate to include the skin borders.

Centring point: with a horizontal central ray 5 cm above the left external auditory meatus.

Radiographic Anatomy

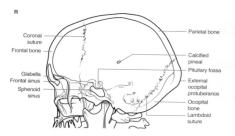

R

Coronal suture
Frontal bone
Glabella
Frontal sinus
Sphenoid sinus

Parietal bone
Calcified pineal
Pituitary fossa
External occipital protuberance
Occipital bone
Lambdoid suture

FIGURE 8.8   Anatomy of the right lateral projection of the skull.

Resultant Image

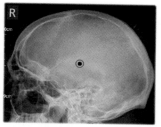

FIGURE 8.9   Resultant image of the right lateral projection of the skull.

Common positioning faults:

Additional projections:

Other notes:

Occipito-mental (OM) Projection of the Facial Bones

Common Indications for Imaging

- Facial bone fractures
- Location of foreign body
- Postoperative assessment of facial bone surgery

Radiographic Technique

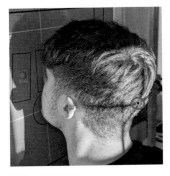

FIGURE 8.10   Patient positioning for the OM projection of the facial bones.

- Sit the patient erect in a chair.
- Raise the patient's chin and rest it against the IR.
- Ensure that the radiographic baseline is at 45° to the floor.
- Ensure that the interpupillary line is parallel to the floor.
- Ensure that the median sagittal plane is perpendicular to the IR.
- Ensure that the patient is not rotated.
- Place the anatomical marker in the primary beam.
- Collimate to include the skin borders.

Centring point: with a horizontal central ray in the midline so that the central ray exits at the level of the lower orbital margin.

Radiographic Anatomy

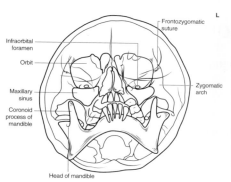

FIGURE 8.11 Anatomy of the OM projection of the facial bones.

Resultant Image

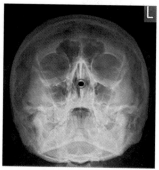

FIGURE 8.12 Resultant image of the OM projection of the facial bones.

Common positioning faults:

Additional projections:

Other notes:

Occipito-mental (OM) 30° Projection of the Facial Bones

Common Indications for Imaging

- Facial bone fractures
- Location of foreign body
- Postoperative assessment of facial bone surgery

Radiographic Technique

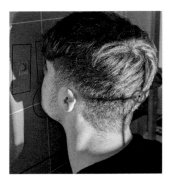

FIGURE 8.13 Patient positioning for the OM 30° projection of the facial bones.

- Sit the patient erect in a chair.
- Raise the patient's chin and rest it against the IR.
- Ensure that the radiographic baseline is at 45° to the floor.
- Ensure that the interpupillary line is parallel to the floor.
- Ensure that the median sagittal plane is perpendicular to the IR.
- Ensure that the patient is not rotated.
- Place the anatomical marker in the primary beam.
- Collimate to include the skin borders.

Centring point: with a horizontal central ray angled 30° caudally in the midline so that the central ray exits at the level of the symphysis menti.

Radiographic Anatomy

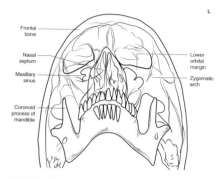

FIGURE 8.14 Anatomy of the OM 30° projection of the facial bones.

Labels on Figure 8.14:
- Frontal bone
- Nasal septum
- Maxillary sinus
- Coronoid process of mandible
- Lower orbital margin
- Zygomatic arch

Resultant Image

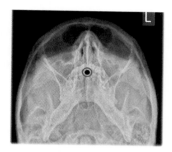

FIGURE 8.15 Resultant image of the OM 30° projection of the facial bones.

Common positioning faults:

Additional projections:

Other notes:

Lateral Projection of the Facial Bones (Right)

Common Indications for Imaging

- Facial bone fractures
- Location of foreign body
- Postoperative assessment of facial bone surgery

Radiographic Technique

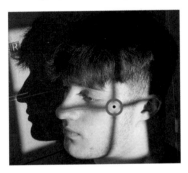

FIGURE 8.16 Patient positioning for the right lateral projection of the facial bones.

- Sit the patient erect in a chair.
- Turn the patient so that the right side of their head is in contact with the IR.
- Ensure that the radiographic baseline is parallel to the floor.
- Ensure that the interpupillary line is parallel to the floor.
- Ensure that the median sagittal plane is parallel to the IR.
- Ensure that the patient is not rotated.
- Place the right anatomical marker in the primary beam.
- Collimate to include the skin borders.

Centring point: with a horizontal central ray at a point 2.5 cm inferior to the outer canthus of the left eye.

Radiographic Anatomy

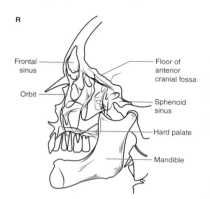

R

Frontal sinus

Orbit

Floor of anterior cranial fossa

Sphenoid sinus

Hard palate

Mandible

FIGURE 8.17   Anatomy of the right lateral projection of the facial bones.

Resultant Image

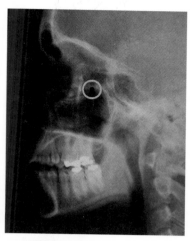

FIGURE 8.18   Resultant image of the right lateral projection of the facial bones.

Common positioning faults:

Additional projections:

Other notes:

Postero-anterior (PA) Projection of the Mandible

Common Indications for Imaging

- Mandible fractures
- Postoperative assessment of mandibular surgery

Radiographic Technique

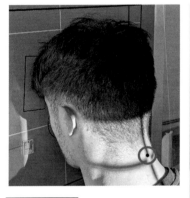

FIGURE 8.19   Patient positioning for the PA projection of the mandible.

- Sit the patient erect in a chair.
- Rest the patient's forehead and nose against the IR.
- Ensure that the radiographic baseline is parallel to the floor.
- Ensure that the interpupillary line is parallel to the floor.
- Ensure that the median sagittal plane is perpendicular to the IR.
- Ensure that the patient is not rotated.
- Place the anatomical marker in the primary beam.
- Collimate to include the temperomandibular joints superiorly, the symphysis menti inferiorly and laterally the skin borders

Centring point: with a horizontal central ray midway so that the central ray exits between the temperomandibular joints and the symphysis menti in the midline (at the philtrum).

Radiographic Anatomy

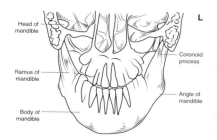

Head of mandible
Coronoid process
Ramus of mandible
Angle of mandible
Body of mandible
L

FIGURE 8.20   Anatomy of the PA projection of the mandible.

Resultant Image

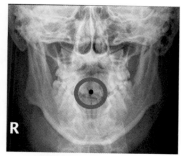

R

FIGURE 8.21   Resultant image of the PA projection of the mandible.

Common positioning faults:

Additional projections:

Other notes:

Lateral Oblique Projections of the Mandible (Right)

Common Indications for Imaging

- Mandible fractures
- Postoperative assessment of mandibular surgery

Radiographic Technique

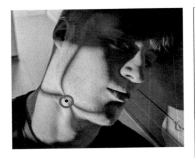

FIGURE 8.22 Patient positioning for the left lateral oblique projection of the mandible.

- Sit the patient erect in a chair.
- Turn the patient so that the right side of their head is in contact with the IR.
- Adjust the patient's head to an oblique position so that the median sagittal plane is at 30° to the IR.
- Ensure that the patient is not rotated.
- Place the right anatomical marker in the primary beam.
- Collimate to include the mandible.
- Both sides are taken for comparison, so a left lateral oblique with the left side of the patient's head in contact with IR should follow.

Centring point: with a horizontal central ray 5 cm below the angle of the mandible distant from the IR, in this case the left.

Radiographic Anatomy

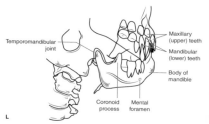

Temporomandibular joint
Maxillary (upper) teeth
Mandibular (lower) teeth
Body of mandible
Coronoid process
Mental foramen
L

FIGURE 8.23   Anatomy of the left lateral oblique projection of the mandible.

Resultant Image

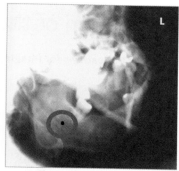

FIGURE 8.24   Resultant image of the left lateral oblique projection of the mandible.

Common positioning faults:

Additional projections:

Other notes:

Occipito-frontal (OF) 20° Projection of the Orbits

Common Indications for Imaging

- Foreign bodies in the orbits, before undergoing magnetic resonance imaging

Radiographic Technique

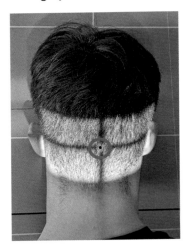

FIGURE 8.25 Patient positioning for the OF 20° projection of the orbits.

- Sit the patient erect in a chair.
- Rest the patient's forehead and nose against the IR.
- Ensure that the radiographic baseline is parallel to the floor.
- Ensure that the interpupillary line is parallel to the floor.
- Ensure that the median sagittal plane is perpendicular to the IR.
- Ensure that the patient is not rotated.
- Place the anatomical marker in the primary beam.
- Collimate to include the superior and inferior borders of the orbits.
- One projection should be taken with the patient looking up (eyes up) and one with the patient looking down (eyes down).

Centring point: with a horizontal central ray angled 20° caudally in the midline with the beam exiting at the nasion.

Radiographic Anatomy

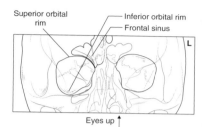

Superior orbital rim

Inferior orbital rim

Frontal sinus

L

Eyes up ↑

FIGURE 8.26   Anatomy of the OF 20° projection of the orbits.

Resultant Image

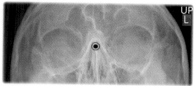

UP
L

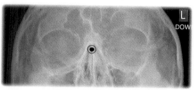

L
DOW

FIGURE 8.27   Resultant image of the OF 20° projection of the orbits – eyes up and eyes down.

Common positioning faults:

Additional projections:

Other notes:

Dental Panoramic Tomography (DPT)

Common Indications for Imaging

- Orthodontic assessment
- Presence and position of wisdom teeth
- Periodontal disease and alveolar bone levels
- Site and size of lesions in the mandible – cysts, tumours
- Diseases of the maxillary sinuses
- Assessment of temporomandibular joints
- Fractures of the mandible

Radiographic Technique

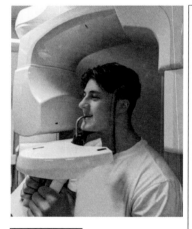

FIGURE 8.28 Patient positioning for the DPT.

- Stand the patient erect.
- The median sagittal plane should be perpendicular to the floor.
- Feet apart, to give a stable base.
- The Frankfurt plane should be parallel to the floor.
- The patient should be placed in the machine using the head-positioning devices and light-beam markers.
- The anterior incisors should be occluded onto the bite block.
- There is normally a vertical light to align to the 2/3 interdental space.
- Patients should place their tongue into the roof of their mouth.
- Patients should close their lips.

Centring point: the DPT has an automatic centring device, so it is important that the patient is positioned accurately.

Radiographic Anatomy

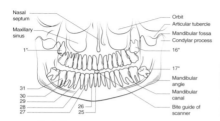

Nasal
septum
Maxillary
sinus
1*
31
30
29
28
27

26
25

Orbit
Articular tubercle
Mandibular fossa
Condylar process
16*

17*
Mandibular
angle
Mandibular
canal
Bite guide of
scanner

FIGURE 8.29   Anatomy of the DPT.

Resultant Image

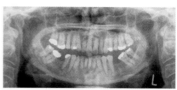

FIGURE 8.30   Resultant image of the DPT.

Common positioning faults:

Additional projections:

Other notes:

Index

Fundamentals of Radiographic Positioning and Anatomy, First Edition.
Jane M. Harvey-Lloyd, Ruth M. Strudwick and Scott J. Preston.
© 2025 John Wiley & Sons Ltd. Published 2025 by John Wiley & Sons Ltd.